RC
425
.A63
1980

ANGELO STATE UNIVERSITY

3 0000 000 622 245

Aphasia

Aphasia

Assessment and Treatment

EDITORS

MARTHA TAYLOR SARNO

Department of Rehabilitation Medicine,
New York University School of Medicine, USA

OLLE HÖÖK

Institute of Rehabilitation Medicine,
Sahlgren's Hospital, Göteborg, Sweden

WITHDRAWN

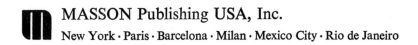 MASSON Publishing USA, Inc.

New York · Paris · Barcelona · Milan · Mexico City · Rio de Janeiro

© 1980 by
Almqvist & Wiksell International,
Stockholm, Sweden

No part of this publication may be reproduced or
transmitted in any form, or by any means, electronic
or mechanical, including photocopy, recording, or any
information storage and retrieval system, without
permission in writing from the copyright owner.

First published by
Almqvist & Wiksell International
Stockholm/Sweden
ISBN 91-22-00388-6

in collaboration with

Masson Publishing USA, Inc.
New York
ISBN 0-89352-086-1
Library of Congress Catalog Card
Number 80-80488

Martha Taylor Sarno – Olle Höök. APHASIA. Assessment
and Treatment. Reports from a joint symposium of the
Research Committees on Aphasia and on Neurological
Rehabilitation of the World Federation of Neurology.

Printed in Sweden by
Almqvist & Wiksell, Uppsala 1980

Contents

Contributors

Frank Benson, M.D.
Neurobehavioral Center
Boston Veterans Administration
  Medical Center
Department of Neurology
Boston Univ. School of Medicine
Boston, Mass., USA

Arthur L. Benton, Ph.D.
Department of Neurology
University Hospitals
Iowa City, IA 52242, USA

Gunnar Bjuggren, M.D.
Emanuel Birkes väg 6
S-144 00 Rönninge, Sweden

Hans M. Borchgrevink, M.D.
Institute of Aviation Medicine
P.O. Box 281
N-Blindern-Oslo 3, Norway

Ingrid Braminder, Speech Therapist
Sundbyberg Hospital
Järnvägsgatan 25
S-172 37 Sundbyberg, Sweden

Antonio R. Damasio, M.D., Director
Division of Behavioral Neurology
University of Iowa College of Medicine
Iowa City, IA 52242, USA

Ennio De Renzi, M.D., Professor
Department of Neurology
Policlinico Universitario
Via del Pozzo 71
Modena 41100, Italy

A. Duval, Linguist
U.E.R. Langage
Université de Haute-Bretagne
Avenue Gaston Berger
F-35000 Rennes, France

Harald Engvik
Department of Psychology
University of Oslo
N-Oslo, Norway

J. Gagnepain, Professor
U.E.R. Langage
Université de Haute-Bretagne
Avenue Gaston Berger
F-35000 Rennes, France

H. Guyard, Linguist
U.E.R. Langage
Université de Haute-Bretagne
Avenue Gaston Berger
F-35000 Rennes, France

W. Huber, Ph.D.
Neurolinguistics
Abteilung Neurologie
Rheinisch-Westfälische Technische
  Hochschule
Goethestrasse 27/29
BRD-51 Aachen, West-Germany

Olle Höök, M.D., Professor
Institute of Rehabilitation Medicine
Sahlgren's Hospital
Övre Husargatan 36
S-413 14 Göteborg, Sweden

Eva Ihre, Speech Therapist
Department of Phoniatrics
Huddinge Hospital
S-141 86 Huddinge, Sweden

Keith Knox, B.Sc.
Department, L.M.C.
Royal Institute of Technology
S-100 44 Stockholm 70, Sweden

Kristian Kristiansen, M.D., Professor
Department of Neurosurgery
Ullevål sykehus
N-Oslo 1, Norway

Bo Larsen, M.D.
Department of Clinical Physiology
Bispebjerg Hospital
DK-Copenhagen NV, Denmark

Yvan Lebrun, Ph.D., Professor
Neurolinguistics
Akademisch Ziekenhuis V.U.B.
Laarbeeklaan
B-1090 Brussels, Belgium

André Roch Lecours, M.D.
Centre de rééducation du langage et de
  recherche neuropsychologique
Hôtel-Dieu de Montréal
3840 rue Saint-Urbain
Montréal H2W 1T8, Québec, Canada

Stina Linell, Speech Therapist
Institute of Rehabilitation Medicine
Sahlgren's Hospital
Övre Husargatan 36
S-413 14 Göteborg, Sweden

Ellen Osborn
Escola Paulista de Medicina
Sao Paulo, Brasil

Klaus Poeck, M. D., Professor
Abteilung Neurologie
Rheinisch-Westfälische Technische
  Hochschule
Goethestrasse 27/29
BRD-51 Aachen, West Germany

Ivar Reinvang, Psychologist
Institute for Aphasia and Stroke
Sunnaas Hospital
N-1450 Nesoddtangen, Norway

Olivier Sabouraud, M.D., Professor
Service de Neurologie
Centre Hospitalier & Universitaire de
  Rennes
Bloc Hopital de Pontchaillou
Rue Henri le Guilloux
F-35043 Rennes, France

Leena Salonen, B.A., D.T.S.T.
Department of Neurosurgery
Helsinki University Central Hospital
Topeliuksenkatu 5
SF-00260 Helsinki, Finland

Martha Taylor Sarno, Professor
Department of Rehabilitation Medicine
New York University School of Medicine
400 East 34th Street
New York, N.Y. 10016, USA

Sumiko Sasanuma, Ph.D., Professor
Yokohama National University
156 Tokiwadai, Hodogaya-Ku
Yokohama – 240, Japan

Erik Skinhøj, M.D., Professor
Department of Neurology
Rigshospitalet
DK-2100 Copenhagen, Denmark

Franz-Josef Stachowiak, Ph.D.
Neurolinguistics
Abteilung Neurologie
Rheinisch-Westfälische Technische
  Hochschule
Goethestrasse 27/29
BRD-51 Aachen, West-Germany

Göran Steg, M.D., Professor
Department of Neurology
University of Göteborg
Sahlgren's Hospital
S-413 45 Göteborg, Sweden

Inger Vibeke Thomsen, M.D., Speech
  Pathologist
Department of Neurology
Rigshospitalet
DK-2100 Copenhagen, Denmark

Lisa Travis
Department of Linguistics
McGill University
Montreal, Canada

Dorothea Weniger, Ph.D.
Neurolinguistics
Abteilung Neurologie
Rheinisch-Westfälische Technische
  Hochschule
Goethestrasse 27/29
BRD-51 Aachen, West-Germany

List of Abbreviations

ADL	Activities of Daily Living	MTDDA	Minnesota Test for the Differential Diagnosis of Aphasia
Amerind	American Indian Sign Language	NCCEA	Neurosensory Center Comprehensive Examination for Aphasia
BDAE	Boston Diagnostic Aphasia Examination	NF	Non-Fluent
CADL	Communication Abilities of Daily Living	PICA	Porch Index of Communicative Ability
CAT Scan or CT Scan	Computerized Axial Tomography	PST	Phonemic Segmentation Test
CVA	Cerebrovascular Accident	PTA	Post-traumatic Amnesia
EEG	Electroencephalogram	RT	Reporter's Test
F	Fluent	SR	Sentence Repetition
FCP	Functional Communication Profile	TT	Token Test
FLS	Functional Life Scale	UL	Utterance Length
G	Global	VF	Verbal Fluency
IQ	Intelligence Quotient	VIC	Visual Communication Therapy
MIT	Melodic Intonation Therapy	VN	Visual Naming
MLA	Multi Language Aphasia Examination	VOT	Voice Onset Time
		WAB	Western Aphasia Battery
		WPM	Words per minute

Preface

This volume contains the majority of papers presented at the International Symposium on Aphasia sponsored by the Institute of Rehabilitation Medicine, Department of Neurology, and the Department of Phoniatry of the University of Göteborg and held in Göteborg, Sweden in September 1977. The Symposium was supported by the Swedish Medical Research Council, the Swedish Multiple Sclerosis Society, and Folksam.

The conference consisted of a two-day teaching seminar covering four major areas of aphasia recovery and rehabilitation: research, assessment, treatment, and the training of the aphasia therapist, and a two-day joint meeting of the Research Committees on Aphasia and on Neurologic Rehabilitation of the World Federation of Neurology.

The didactic material which was prepared and presented by Martha Taylor Sarno is clustered at the beginning of Part I in order to keep it separate from the individual papers. The selected papers from the World Federation of Neurology committee sessions appear in Part II and are organized according to their order of program presentation.

Göteborg and New York, December 1979

Olle Höök   *Martha Taylor Sarno*

Part I

Martha Taylor Sarno

1. Review of Research in Aphasia
   —Recovery and Rehabilitation

2. Analyzing Aphasic Behavior

3. Aphasia Rehabilitation

Review of research in aphasia: recovery and rehabilitation

MARTHA TAYLOR SARNO

The topic of recovery and rehabilitation in the aphasia literature has received relatively little research attention. This is in part undoubtedly the result of the many problems inherent in studying these aspects of aphasia. An over-riding concern with pathophysiology which has traditionally dominated medical research in chronic diseases has generally stimulated a greater interest in localization and classification. There has also been an attitude of relative indifference on the part of the medical community toward recovery in aphasia perhaps related to the notion that questions concerning recovery and rehabilitation have already been answered (21, 54).

The notion that there was "... sufficient evidence that 're-education' is a valuable means to re-establish man's noblest prerogative—the faculty of articulate language" was suggested by a neurologist as early as 1890 (4). A few years later, another neurologist, Dr Charles K. Mills described the case of a 45-year-old physician with a right hemiplegia and complete aphasia after stroke whom he "retrained" through the use of a pedagogically oriented regimen reminiscent of many speech therapy approaches in current use (43).

In earlier times, aphasia and its concomitant neurological deficits were viewed as a natural and necessary stage in the process of dying. Few expected care and "treatment" was non-existent. In direct contrast, the public today, especially in the industrialized parts of the world assumes the right to medical care and treatment regardless of social or economic status. Along with this, many believe in the magic that "modern" medicine can somehow cure most ills.

The climate of unrealistic expectation which created such an unprecedented demand for services was probably fostered in large part by a diametric expansion of communication and the explosive growth of mass media over the last three decades. Societies became more socially conscious. Whereas chronic disease was previously considered almost taboo, it became a ready subject for public discussion.

The present era of increased therapeutic expectations has led to subsidized medical care. As the cost of such medical care in the United States is rising precipitiously, it becomes imperative that funds used to rehabilitate aphasics be spent wisely.

These changing attitudes and a more vocal lay press in the United States have sharpened the focus on public figures who incurred strokes. Sir Winston

Churchill's stroke in 1953, followed by Present Dwight D. Eisenhower's in 1957 and Ambassador Joseph Kennedy's in 1962 gave the public greater freedom to discuss these incidents. Immediately following General Eisenhower's stroke a series of front page articles written by Eugene J. Taylor, a medical writer long associated with Dr Howard A. Rusk, appeared in the New York Times. Their purpose was a description of aphasia in lay terms.

Several informational booklets designed for use by the families and friends of aphasic patients (1, 2, 5, 51, 65) appeared during the same period. Another book *Understanding Aphasia*, now over twenty years old and translated into eight languages, is still widely read in its original version (65). Workbooks, manuals and other treatment guides for home use were also published (35, 68, 69), as well as personal accounts written by individuals who were aphasic after strokes (8, 26, 47, 74).

In the present decade the emergence of other booklets (60), workbooks (6, 28, 64) and personal accounts (10, 13, 44, 75) attests to a continuing public interest in aphasia.

Although the exact incidence of aphasia in the United States is unknown, present estimates suggest a reservoir of about one million aphasics. The overwhelming majority are those with aphasia secondary to stroke. According to current approximations, roughly 400,000 new strokes occur in the United States each year, at least 84,000 (21 %) of these are accompanied by aphasia, and at 4 to 12 weeks post stroke 10,000 (2.5 %) of these still have severe language disturbances (7).

The rapidly increasing worldwide geriatric population makes it essential that we give serious and careful thought to the topic of aphasia recovery and rehabilitation. A recent census in the United States reported that almost 22 million people were over the age of 65 and it is projected that there will be nearly 31 million persons in this group by the year 2000.[1] The median age for large samples of aphasic stroke patients has been reported as 60 (59), slightly above 65 (52) and 64 (7).

Those engaged in the care of aphasics find themselves in an uncomfortable situation. Circumstances have created a demand for services, yet the factors influencing the recovery and rehabilitation of aphasia are still not well understood. In spite of this, many thousands of aphasic patients have been "treated", many techniques tried, and many speech pathologists trained to treat aphasic patients (66).

The problem associated with designing and conducting research that carefully controls all of the variables which contribute to the recovery process in aphasia are of such magnitude that many investigators have withdrawn from research in this area. The important variables of age, etiology, size and site of lesion, type and severity of aphasia, time since onset and educational level have been thoroughly discussed by various authors (14, 15, 18, 55, 71).

---

[1] Current Population Report U.S. Census Bureau. P. 25, No. 541, February 1975.

In addition to the many problems mentioned in the literature a significant and seemingly universal problem in aphasia is the lack of a uniform classification and description of the patient with aphasia. It remains virtually impossible to compare the results of any studies dealing with recovery or treatment because of differences in emphasis, modes of reporting, and lack of a common nomenclature. A term such as "recovery" is often used when partial 'improvement' is meant; "loss of language" could mean either 'paucity of utterance', 'lack of comprehension', or 'difficulty in production', etc. "Learning to speak" usually suggests return to a status quo without signs of actual learning or relearning (32).

During the earliest part of the twentieth century the literature is focused more exclusively on clinical observations rather than recovery and rehabilitation of traumatic aphasia, and the record shows clearly that the post-traumatic aphasic enjoys a better outcome than the post-stroke patient, that time since onset and the early initiation of speeeh therapy enhance recovery and that younger patients fare best (9, 16, 73). Those who have attempted retraining have almost without exception, reported it to be effective. Some representative summaries of earlier reports of findings obtained on post-traumatic patients follow.

Franz (19) and Head (25) reported recovery and reeducation findings on limited samples of aphasic patients primarily the result of missile wounds. Goldstein observed 90 to 100 aphasic patients across a 10 year period in Frankfurt during World War I and emphasized the more favorable outcome of the patients with aphasia resulting from missile wound when compared to aphasia secondary to apoplexy. He concluded that retraining had an important influence on recovery in the post-missile wound aphasic and that improvement beyond spontanous recovery requires special effort on the patient's part which he may not be able to achieve without help. Goldstein felt that successful retraining demanded great effort, skill and time (22). Granich (23) and Eisenson (16) also reported their experiences in reeducating combat soldiers with missile wounds.

In another early study, Butfield and Zangwill (9) followed 66 aphasic patients, the majority of whom were post-trauma. After re-education, speech was judged to be significantly improved, both in patients who began therapy less than 6 months after onset (half of group) and more than 6 months after onset (third of group). In oral speech production, 46 % of the total group (mostly young adults) were judged "much improved"; 31 % were "improved"; and 23 % were "unimproved". Of the patients who were treated less than 6 months post onset, 40 % were "much improved" while only 22 % of the group who were treated after 6 months post onset were judged as "much improved".

The work of Russell and Espir (49) and Teuber (70) did not address itself specifically to concerns of recovery and rehabilitation but made classic contributions to the literature on aphasia after missile wounds.

Luria has provided detailed descriptions of his rationales for therapy as well as explicit examples of cases and techniques based on extensive experience with traumatic aphasic patients (37, 39, 40). He believed that systematic retraining based on a careful analysis of the psycholinguistic breakdown and aimed at compensatory function provides the foundation for successful restoration of verbal activities.

One of the first comprehensive reports of retraining aphasic World War II veterans on a large scale was that of Wepman (73). He described a group of 68 aphasic patients with a mean age of 25.8 years who began treatment six months post-trauma. Wepman utilized training methods modeled after traditional language educational techniques. He concluded that aphasia following brain trauma is amenable to improvement with training. Specifically, he found that the expressive aphasic group recovered the highest levels of language performance followed by receptive and global groups of aphasics, in that order.

Certain studies in the English language literature have concerned themselves with recovery in aphasic patients who are primarily post-stroke. There is a general lack of equivalence among studies. The Marks, Taylor and Rusk (41) and Vignolo (71) studies, for example, addressed themselves specifically to the question of outcome in recovery from aphasia.

Marks, Taylor and Rusk (41) studied 203 aphasic patients who were treated in a rehabilitation setting; 93 % of the group had suffered strokes. Rehabilitation outcome was based primarily on clinical judgements about whether patients moved from lower to higher diagnostic or functional groups. Functional categories ranged from the lowest level (institutional adequacy) to the highest (vocational adequacy). The results of this study supported the idea that there is significant functional benefit to be derived for patients who are exposed to comprehensive language training in a rehabilitation setting, especially those with expressive aphasia.

In a retrospective study of 69 patients Vignolo (71) categorized patients into two groups: 42 patients who received speech therapy and 27 who were untreated. He concluded that there is a spontaneous evolution in the direction of recovery of function and that re-education had a specific effect as long as it lasted more than six months. The receptive aspect tends to improve more than expression. In his study, the initial level of auditory comprehension did not influence improvement in oral expression. Time since onset emerged as an important prognostic factor: two and six months from onset seem to be important milestones in recovery.

In the study of 30 treated post-stroke aphasic patients by Sands, Sarno and Shankweiler (50) improvement in language function was measured by the *Functional Communication Profile* (FCP) (53, 67), a functional rating scale. The median gain for all patients was ten percentage points. Only three patients did not improve. Age appeared to be the most important variable influencing recovery.

In another study (57) 31 patients who were at least three months post-stroke and classified as alert global aphasics were randomly assigned to three treatment conditions: programmed instruction, "traditional" speech therapy and no treatment. Though equated for time since onset the sample was widely heterogeneous, with some patients up to ten years post-stroke. All patients showed small gains but there were no significant differences in gains for any of the groups. The results of this study supported the clinical impression that global aphasics show minimal but not significant improvement, with or without therapy, an opinion already expressed by Schuell (59).

Smith (61, 62) studied 80 relatively young (mean age of 51.3 years) treated aphasic patients. Sixty-seven patients had a vascular etiology and 13 patients were post-traumatic. Moderate or marked improvement in speech was noted in 55 % of the group, in comprehension 67 %, in reading 61 %, and in writing 54 % was exhibited.

Hagen (24) studied the effects of treatment in 20 males with communication disorders after stroke, with a mean age of 52.6 years. Ten patients received therapy for one year while the other group did not. Although both groups exhibited spontaneous improvement during the first three months, only the treatment group of patients receiving treatment continued to improve beyond what is generally considered the spontaneous recovery period.

The positive effect of treatment on oral expression, even if undertaken six months after onset of aphasia was reported by Basso et al. (3). One hundred and eighty-five subjects were studied; 91 receiving therapy (three sessions per week for six consecutive months) and 94 not re-educated. The mean age of the group was 48.1 years and aphasia was the result of vascular, non-progressive lesions in the majority of patients. (Both Wernicke's and Broca's aphasics were studied.) In addition, Basso et al. found that the longer the time since onset, the less progress is likely.

Rose et al. (48) studied 50 patients referred for speech therapy (mean age of 65.7 years) and 21 patients who were not referred (mean age of 65.6 years). The only positive relationship with improvement was the number of hours of treatment. Other factors suggested as prognostic indicators included sex, age, hemiplegia, speech diagnosis, length of stay in hospital; however, none were found to be of significance.

More recently Kertesz and McCabe (30) reported findings on 93 post CVA aphasics in whom they controlled for time since onset. The degree of improvement was greatest in the period between $1\frac{1}{2}$ months post-stroke and three months post-stroke. Both untreated global aphasics and anomics improved less than Broca's aphasics with respect to rate of improvement but not degree of improvement. There was a high correlation between initial severity and outcome. No correlation was found between rate of recovery and age. In addition, they found the younger the patient, the higher the initial recovery rate; traumatic aphasics had a better overall prognosis than vascular disease; and that almost all globals remained poor. Where such a comparison was possible, no significant differences were found between treated and untreated patient groups.

Levita (33) compared *Functional Communication Profile* (53, 67) results for 17 treated and 18 untreated aphasic patients. All treated patients received therapy during the period between four and 12 seeks post-onset. No significant differences were found between the groups. Results suggest that patients who received traditional speech therapy could not be differentiated from untreated controls.

What is perhaps the most important concern related to previous studies on recovery is that they have been done, for the most part, on populations dissimilar from one which demands our attention today: the post-stroke, older patient.

Although Weisenberg and McBride (71) concerned themselves with the general topic of aphasia, without special reference to recovery, their five year study did provide some minimal information on recovery and re-education. There were 60 patients of less than 60 years of age, and the majority had suffered strokes. This was one of the first studies which used standardized psychological measures as a basis for their findings. The authors concluded that re-education not only increased the rate of recovery but assists in facilitating the use of compensatory means of communication and improves morale.

Based on extensive experiences in the rehabilitation of aphasics at the Minneapolis Veterans Administration Hospital, the majority of whom were post-stroke, the late Hildred Schuell believed that selected types of aphasia recovered under a therapeutic approach which emphasized psychological support and carefully controlled auditory stimulation. She stressed the necessity for controlling the complexity, length, rate and loudness of stimulation (58, 59). Since World War II, certain issues in the study of recovery and rehabilitation in aphasia have been brought into sharper focus and new questions have been raised. Furthermore, our knowledge about some of the factors which influence recovery and rehabilitation has been increased in important ways. Some of this new knowledge is the result of findings concerning the characterization of spontaneous recovery.

Spontaneous recovery

In his studies of the post-traumatic aphasic, Luria referred to a period of six to seven months post-onset as the time when spontaneous restitution might take place. 43 % of his group showed residual signs requiring re-education or psychotherapy after that period (38). In a group of 21 untreated post-stroke aphasic patients Culton (11) found that rapid spontaneous recovery of language function was noted in the first months following the onset of aphasia as well as spontaneous recovery of intellectual function. These increases were not evident in the second month post-onset.

Sarno and Levita (55) studied 28 untreated post-stroke patients with severe aphasia in the first six months post-stroke and found that greater change took place within a three month than a six month post period.

Brust et al. (7) surveyed 850 acute (first month post) stroke patients during a three year period. Aphasia was present in 177 patients (21 % of group) during the acute phase; 32 % were classified as Fluent and 68 % as Non-Fluent. In the Non-Fluent group of 120 patients, 35 were mild and 72 were global. In the period 4–12 weeks post-stroke, the aphasia improved in 74 % of the patients and cleared in 44 %. At three months post-stroke, 12 % in the Fluent group and 34 % in the Non-Fluent group were still considered impaired. These findings add to our understanding of the nature of the spontaneous recovery period. Clearly, the patient with Fluent aphasia in the first month post-stroke has a better chance of improving before the end of the spontaneous recovery period.

Lomas and Kertesz (34) tested 31 aphasic stroke patients within 30 days (mean of 11.5 days) and at three months (mean of 97 days) post-stroke. Eight language tests (i.e., yes/no responses, repetition, imitation, naming, Token Test, spontaneous speech in picture description and conversational questions) were administered. There was a great variation in amount of improvement; not all improved to the same degree. The low fluency/low comprehension patients made the least recovery, and the low fluency/high comprehension patients the most. Initial comprehension proved to be a good prognostic indicator. (Lomas said "Perhaps Schuell was right.")

The influence of therapy

All of the studies of the effects of therapy on aphasia have, virtually without exception, concluded that language training has a positive effect on outcome. None of the studies is definitive and the overwhelming number did not include an untreated control group. Furthermore, most studies used patients with mixed etiologies. In general, the differences among studies with respect to controlling variables such as time since onset, criteria for "improvement" and other problems of research design makes our knowledge of the efficacy of treatment very limited.

Age and recovery

While there is little disagreement as to the more favorable prognosis of the patient with post-traumatic aphasia (9, 17, 18, 21, 30, 38, 73) there is little consensus with respect to the influence of age.

Vignolo (71), Gerstman and Woodbury (20) and Sands et al. (50) concluded that the younger patient recovered to a greater degree. Vignolo placed 69 aphasic patients into three age categories: young (less than 40 years), middle-aged (40–60 years), and old (more than 60 years) and found more than 70 % of the young group improved, yet only 22 % of the older group improved.

In a study of 30 treated aphasic patients with a mean age of 56.5 years, age appeared to be the most potent variable influencing recovery (50). The prognosis for a good recovery was much better for patients less than 50 years of age than those over 60. The sixth of the total group which showed the greatest improvement were found to be the youngest patients (average of 47 years) while the sixth which showed the least improvement averaged 61 years of age.

In contrast, Culton (12), Sarno and Levita (55), Smith (61, 62), Rose et al. (48), Messerli et al. (42) and Kertesz and McCabe (30) reported no correlation between recovery and age.

Type of aphasia and recovery

In the recent study of Kertesz and McCabe (30) Broca's aphasics had the highest rate of recovery. The lowest rate of recovery occurred within the global aphasic group. Lomas and Kertesz (34) reported significant differences in recovery between different types of aphasia during the first three months post-stroke.

There were no qualitative or quantitative differences between groups (Fluent, Mixed, Non-Fluent, Severely Non-Fluent) despite the differences in severity in the study reported by Prins et al. (45). Using fluency alone as the basis for classification, there was a lack of differentiation between any type of aphasia. Even though fluency had a high correlation with degree of severity the pattern of change over the course of one year, that is, the relatively greater improvement in comprehension than spontaneous speech, was the same for all types of aphasia.

Severity and recovery

No investigator has reported that the more severe aphasias recover as well as milder forms. Schuell et al. (59) found severity of aphasia to be associated with a predictable pattern of recovery. Sands et al. (50) evaluated 30 patients pre- and post-treatment on the *Functional Communication Profile* and concluded that the severity of language impairment at initial evaluation is a moderately good predictor of the amount of recovery that may be expected. This was verified by Sarno et al. (57) who studied severe aphasic patients receiving speech therapy and reported only small gains. They improved only on imitative tasks while the mildly impaired improved on all modalities in the study by Kenin and Swisher (29). Kertesz and McCabe (30) also reported that the more severe patients made less improvement.

Global aphasia is generally viewed as a correlate of the least improved (30, 59, 76) except in the case of our own yet unpublished report of systematic observations of patients for one year post-stroke, which showed that although global aphasics never reached the levels of language performance achieved by the fluent and non-fluent groups, they did make greater gains in language tasks in the six months to one year period post-stroke (56). In the Prins study (45) some global aphasic patients were reclassified as non-fluent.

Neuroradiologic correlates of recovery

By examining CAT scans in 14 post CVA aphasic patients during the acute phase and up to eight months, Yarnell et al. (76) concluded that the CAT scan showed a high degree of correlation with aphasia outcome for size, location and number of lesions. Those patients with large dominant hemisphere involvements, either one large or many smaller lesions, fared poorly while those with lesser lesions did better. Bilateral lesions, at times evasive clinically, helped to account for significant aphasia residuals. Fluent aphasics showed predominantly left posteroparietal lesions, whereas, global aphasics showed bilateral, either partly temporal, or large single dominant hemisphere lesions on CAT scan.

Recovery of linguistic rules

A study by Ludlow (36) and another by Reinvang (46) focused on the recovery of syntactic rules.

Ludlow studied 10 treated, five untreated aphasics and five normal controls during the first three months post CVA using a taped sample of free speech and selected language tasks. The measures were administered nine times to each study subject. Analyses included a measurement of sentence length, an index of grammaticality, of sentence production, and a tabulation of transformations. The aphasic patients in this study did not develop a simplified language system in connected speech, but attempted to recover the same structures used premorbidly. The relative frequency of structures was similar to normal speakers. A common pattern of syntactic sequence was observed in the course of recovery for both treated or untreated. Ludlow noted no changes in language competence and concluded that recovery can be interpreted as an increase in the proficiency of language use (language performance). Further, there was no difference in the sequence of recovery with respect to type of aphasia (fluent and non-fluent).

Reinvang (46) studied sentence recovery in two aphasics: a Broca's aphasia secondary to stroke in a 44 year old man, and Wernicke's aphasia in a 73-year-old head injured patient. Findings were based on an analysis of spontaneous speech and tasks of sentence repetition and sentence judgement. Reinvang concluded that syntactically normal utterances were produced with regularity in the patients' speech samples and that an increase in utterance length was a dominant feature in recovery. The main form of deviant utterances were incomplete sentences.

Recovery patterns

The idea that comprehension improves more than expression has been supported by a number of studies (29, 31, 45, 71). Vignolo (71) reported that expressive disturbances were more important than receptive difficulties in preventing the restitution of overall verbal communication. The pattern of recovery for all patient groups over a course of one year was reported to be essentially the same by Prins et al. (45). All groups showed significant improvement in comprehension, however, none showed significant changes in spontaneous speech.

In contrast to these reports the studies by Sarno and Levita (55) and Kertesz and McCabe (30) showed that expression improves more than comprehension.

The many problems inherent in the measurement of auditory comprehension in aphasia will be emphasized in the discussion of the analysis of aphasic behavior. Yet these very problems are associated with a number of apparently conflicting findings extant in the literature.

Time since onset and recovery

Time since onset has received relatively little, specific attention in the aphasic literature. In his retrospective study of the evolution of aphasia, Vignolo (71) reported that as the time interval from onset increased, the number of patients improving decreased. Patients who received training for more than and less than six months were studied; and findings showed that the long term group improved to a greater degree. When considering treatment beginning up to two months and after four months post-stroke, Sands et al. (50) reported greater improvement in the earlier treatment group. The influence of early treatment on gains in language function were also demonstrated in Smith's (62) study. Changes after the first year post-stroke were noted by Marks et al. (41) and Sands et al. (50). On the other hand, Kertesz and McCabe (30) reported little or no change after the first year.

The importance of time since onset has been emphasized recently in three comprehensive recovery studies: Kertesz and McCabe (30), Prins et al. (45) and Sarno and Levita (56). The findings in these studies point to the necessity for taking account of temporal factors in studies of recovery and rehabilitation in aphasia. In the study by Kertesz and McCabe, patients were tested after stroke at four predetermined time intervals: initial test from 0–6 weeks post-onset; followed by retests at three months, six months and yearly intervals.

Prins et al. (45) analyzed, transcribed and scored a taped speech corpus based on a linguistic paradigm, the Token Test, and a sentence comprehension test, on 54 aphasic patients across the first year post CVA. These tests were administered at three specified time intervals (six month intervals) in the course of one year. There was no overall improvement in spontaneous speech in any group, however, all groups did show considerable improvement in sentence comprehension over time.

In our most recent study (56) we systematically examined 43 treated aphasic patients during the one year post-stroke period. Patients were evenly distributed across Fluent (F), Non-Fluent (NF), and Global (G) categories and had a median age of 58 years. They were a highly educated group (median 13 years). In the four to eight week period, little change was observed on any of the

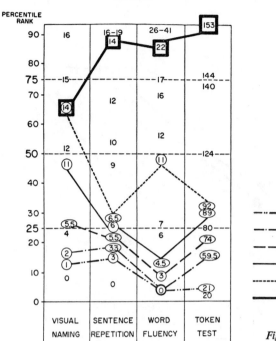

NCCEA

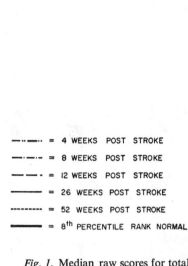

—··—··— = 4 WEEKS POST STROKE

—·—·— = 8 WEEKS POST STROKE

—— —· = 12 WEEKS POST STROKE

———— = 26 WEEKS POST STROKE

·········· = 52 WEEKS POST STROKE

════ = 8th PERCENTILE RANK NORMAL

Fig. 1. Median raw scores for total group.

measures administered. However, in the 12 to 26 week period all diagnostic groups, particularly those designated as F made gains on all measures. The F group made the greatest change on the Token Test (23.5) and the smallest gain on Sentence Repetition (1.5). On the *Functional Communication Profile* (FCP), F patients made a gain on overall score of 11 %.

The group which performed closest to normal at 12 weeks post-stroke was the NF group. At six months post, both F and NF groups, although different in language impairment profiles showed a similar proximity to normal.

In the six to 12 month period the trend toward improvement continued for the whole group on both task performance on NCCEA (63) subtests and functional measures (FCP). (See Figs. 1 and 2.)

In this recovery period the greatest changes on the NCCEA subtests were made by the Global group and the smallest gains by the Fluent group which was the reverse of our findings in the three to six month period. The most remarkable finding for this period was the magnitude of performance improvement on the Token Test achieved by the Global group, a result which supports Kertesz' and McCabe's (30) and Prins et al. (45) studies.

If we look at the all inclusive period from one month to one year, the general trend indicates improvement in all areas. The median overall change on the NCCEA tasks for the whole group across the entire study period was 71 on the Token Test; 11 on Word Fluency; 3.5 on Sentence Repetition; and 13 on

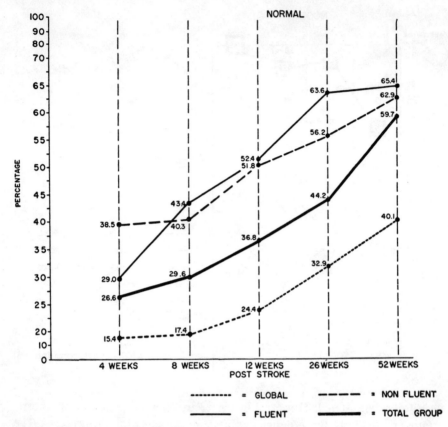

NORMAL

Fig. 2. FCP[1] overall scores (based on median scores by groups).

Visual Naming. The Overall score on the FCP increased by a median of 33.1 points across the year for the total group.

The primary finding of this study was the persistence of improvement in all patients up to one year post-stroke which agrees with the long term reports of other investigators and personal accounts of aphasic patients (13, 44, 50, 61, 71). It should be noted here that individual types of aphasics recovered at different rates.

In spite of the fact that the G aphasic patients showed the greatest improvement in the latter part of the first post-stroke year, they failed to evolve to another type of aphasia by the end of the year, never exceeding a 40% overall FCP score. In contrast to the finding of Lomas and Kertesz (34) and Kertesz and McCabe (30) the group which showed the least change in the three month to one year post-stroke year was the NF category. The fact that the G group had the farthest and the NF group the least to go, does not detract from the substantial gains obtained by the G patients.

---

[1] Functional communication profile (Taylor, 1965, Sarno, 1969).

The discrepancy between changes observed on task oriented performance and functional ratings on patients was striking, that is, it is clear that some of the changes observed in the chronic aphasic can be accounted for by extra-linguistic compensatory mechanisms and not by specific language processing changes alone. In this study, the differences found along different time references in the recovery continuum lend strong support to the consideration of "time since onset" as an extremely important variable in studies of recovery from aphasia.

Psychosocial factors and recovery

No relationship was found between educational levels, occupational status before illness, and recovery by Smith (61) and Sarno et al. (57). In a retrospective study Keenan and Brassell (27) reported that "health, employment. and age had little, if any, prognostic value when compared to comprehension and fluency ...". Rose et al. (48) found sex, length of stay in a hospital, speech diagnosis, or presence of hemiplegia to be of no significance as prognostic factors.

In contradistinction to some of these conclusions, individuals who were employed at the time of stroke performed more adequately than those who were unemployed according to a study by Sarno and Levita (55).

Discussion

Only in recent years has there been sufficient interest in aphasia as a chronic medical and social problem, primarily in the disciplines of rehabilitation medicine, speech pathology, neuropsychology and neurolinguistics, to generate some studies. There are probably not many today who hold the view held by some not too many years ago that we know all we need to know about recovery and rehabilitation in aphasia.

When the effects of treatment (intervention) is added, as another variable to the long list of variables which might contribute to the recovery process, a new set of problems arises: 1) How can one gauge the value of therapy without a clear idea of the course of spontaneous recovery? 2) It is almost impossible to find untreated control patients who are truly comparable (with respect to socioeconomic status, educational level, motivation, etc.) to those who are treated. Yet, there is an urgent need for controlled studies which would investigate the effects of specified, structured therapy on actual language parameters preferably with randomized or matched design to avoid selection bias (30). Without specific delineation of the nature, intensity, duration and quality of therapy, the effects of treatment are not measurable (14). 3) To repeat, there still remains a great need for uniformity in the classification and description of the patient with aphasia; without this it is impossible to generalize the results of any study dealing with recovery or rehabilitation. Terms like *mild, moderate,* and *severe* abound in the literature and are virtually without meaning. By extension the measurement of progress requires standard terms and universally accepted criteria (14, 32, 54). A persistant problem arises from the fact that researchers continue to study populations of patients with dissimilar etiologies with the result that the data and conclusions are essentially meaningless.

Two distinctly different types of studies are needed: One whose purpose it is to elucidate the linguistic-neurological phenomena associated with recovery, along the lines of Reinvang (46), Ludlow (36), and Prins et al. (45) studies, and another should focus on the multifaceted process, better characterized by the term *rehabilitation*, in the person who is aphasic. This is, of course, the key to the distinction: one either addresses oneself to a pathological process or to the ravages of that process in a human being, particularly as this affects adjustments to the disabling symptoms.

In line with this distinction we need to specify and define the meaning of the word "recovery". Does "recovery" simply mean the passage of a certain amount of time after onset (as we tend to use the term "spontaneous recovery") or simply, any degree of "improvement" in any modality at any point in time? Or does the word "recovery" mean, and I would take this view,

> the restitution of communication skills which the patient uses in his daily life for purely social purposes (interacting with others) and for use in controlling his environment. The word recovery must take into account some notion of the patient's premorbid personality, vocation, and social situation since it is the approximation to or restitution of premorbid communication function which constitutes true recovery and is the goal of rehabilitation—not the performance of tasks which are not natural language acts ... not necessarily the increase of points (score) on tests which may or may not reflect an increase of actual communication in real life. In this regard "recovery" refers to the use of natural language, that is, the use of the speech code. In fact, there seems to be a greater concern by researchers for the measurement of performance in spontaneous speech (45).

Yarnell (76) pointed out that despite attempts at subjective and objective evaluation "aphasic recovery encompasses many variables which are difficult to evaluate". In his study the patients with the best recovery outcome reported that they did not feel "fully returned to a premorbid state"—that recovery is a relative term. Recovery has a different meaning to the patient and to the health worker. The majority of patients, no matter how well recovered, never feel normal. Perhaps it is not always valid to talk about "recovery" when referring to groups of aphasics who were not at all similar in their language use before their language impairment, despite the fact that age, type of aphasia, etiology and other variables are deemed equivalent. Perhaps education and socio-economic, cultural and premorbid personality features are more deserving of greater concern and specification in recovery studies.

We also need research along the model of Piaget and others ... studies which do not rely on statistical analyses of groups of aphasics but rather on in depth observations, at the "microscopic" level, of individual, carefully selected patients over long periods of time who are systematically observed and documented in their use of natural language.

In view of the many persons now afflicted with aphasia and the expectation that this number will increase markedly in years to come, recovery and rehabilitation is a high priority research topic. Hopefully, meetings like this one will stimulate new research efforts to help assure that the thousands of aphasics who hope for recovery are not offered false hopes but can depend on reasonable and responsible clinical management.

In a book entitled *The Third Killer*, a British journalist named Guy Wint reported some of his feelings about his post-stroke life and made many perceptive and sensitive remarks about the need for research. This seems like an appropriate time to quote his words on the topic: "The knowledge that research is being actively taken up would have a reviving influence upon those already afflicted. Their cross at present is the knowledge that very little is being done which can hold out for them the prospect of some short cut on the way back to active life, or indeed, can hold for mankind such hope of remedy in the knowledge of the treatment and prevention of the disease. Patients would at least be cheered up to think that, by night and day a battle is being waged on their behalf by many of the best intelligences of medicine. They would get over the sense of being the refuse of human life, cases which can be kept alive but about which nothing effective can be done." (74.)

References

1. Aphasia and the Family. American Heart Association, Publication EM 359, 1969.
2. Backus, O. & Henry, L.: Aphasia in Adults. University of Michigan, Ann Arbor, 1947.
3. Basso, A., Faglione, P. & Vignolo, L.: Étude controlée de la rééducation du language dans l'aphasie: comparaison entre aphasiques traités et nontraités. Rev Neurol (Paris) 131: 607, 1975.
4. Bateman, F.: On Aphasia, a Loss of Speech and the Localization of the Faculty of Articulate Language. (Second Edition.) Churchill, London, 1890.
5. Boone, D.: An Adult Has Aphasia. Interstate Printers and Publishers, Illinois, 1965.
6. Brubaker, S.: Workbook for Aphasia: Exercises for the Re-development of Higher Level Language. Wayne State University Press, Detroit, 1978.
7. Brust, J., Shafer, S., Richter, R. & Bruun, B.: Aphasia in acute stroke. Stroke 7: 167, 1976.
8. Buck, M.: Dysphasia: Professional Guidance for Family and Patient. Prentice-Hall, Englewood Cliffs, N.J., 1968.
9. Butfield, E. & Zangwill, O.: Re-education in aphasia: a review of 70 cases. J Neurol Neurosurg Psychiat 9: 75, 1946.
10. Cameron, C.: A Different Drum. Prentice-Hall, Englewood Cliffs, N.J., 1973.

11. Culton, G.: Spontaneous recovery from aphasia. J Speech Hear Res 12: 825, 1969.
12. Culton, G.: Reaction to age as a factor in chronic aphasia in stroke patients. J Speech Hear Dis 36: 563, 1971.
13. Dahlberg, C. & Jaffee, J.: Stroke: A Physician's Personal Account. W. W. Norton, New York 1977.
14. Darley, F.: The efficacy of language rehabilitation in aphasia. J Speech Hear Dis 37, 1972.
15. Darley, F.: Treatment of acquired aphasia. In: W. J. Friedlander (ed.), Advances in Neurology. Vol. 7, pp. 111. Raven Press, New York, 1975.
16. Eisenson, J.: Prognostic factors related to language rehabilitation in aphasic patients. J Speech Hear Dis 14: 262, 1949.
17. Eisenson, J.: Aphasia: a point of view as to the nature of the disorder and factors that determine prognosis for recovery. Int J Neurol 4: 287, 1964.
18. Eisenson, J.: Adult Aphasia: Assessment and Treatment. Prentice-Hall, Englewood Cliffs, N.J., 1973.
19. Franz, S.: Studies in re-education: the aphasics. J Comp Psychol 4: 349, 1924.
20. Gerstman, L. & Woodbury, M.: Computer prediction of language recovery after stroke. Paper presented at the Sixth International Conference on Medical Electronics and Biological Engineering, Tokyo, 1965.
21. Godfrey, C. & Douglass, E.: The recovery process in aphasia. Canadian Med Assoc J 80: 618, 1959.
22. Goldstein, K.: After-effects of Brain Injuries in War: Their Evaluation and Treatment. Grune & Stratton, New York, 1942.
23. Granich, L. & Prangle, G.: Aphasia: A Guide to Retraining. Grune & Stratton, New York, 1947.
24. Hagen, C.: Communication abilities in hemiplegia: effect of speech therapy. Arch Phys Med Rehab 54: 454, 1973.
25. Head, H.: Aphasia and Kindred Disorders of Speech. Vols. I & II. Hafner, New York, 1963. (First edition: Cambridge University Press, 1926.)
26. Hodgins, E. : Episode. Anthenum, New York, 1964.
27. Keenan, J. & Brassell, E.: A study of factors related to prognosis for individual aphasic patients. J Speech Hear Dis 39: 257, 1974.
28. Keith, R.: Speech and Language Rehabilitation: A Workbook for the Neurologically Impaired. Vols. I & II. Interstate Printers & Publishers, Illinois, 1972, 1977.
29. Kenin, M. & Swisher, L.: A study of pattern of recovery in aphasia. Cortex 8: 56, 1972.
30. Kertesz, A. & McCabe, P.: Recovery patterns and prognosis in aphasia. Brain 100: 1, 1977.
31. Lebrun, Y.: Recovery in polygot aphasics. In: Y. Lebrun & R. Hoops (eds.), Recovery in Aphasics—Neurolinguistics 4, pp. 96–108. Swets & Zeitlinger, B.V., Amsterdam, 1976.
32. Lenneberg, E.: Biological Foundations of Language. Wiley & Sons, New York, 1967.
33. Levita, E. : Effects of speech therapy on aphasics' responses to the Functional Communication Profile. Percep Motor Skills 47: 151, 1978.
34. Lomas, A. & Kertesz, A. : Patterns of spontaneous recovery in aphasic groups: a study of adult stroke patients. Brain Lang 5: 388, 1978.
35. Longerich, M. & Bordeaux, J.: Aphasia Therapeutics. Macmillan, New York, 1954.
36. Ludlow, C.: Recovery from aphasia: a foundation for treatment. In: M. Sullivan & M. Krommers (eds.), Rationale for Adult Aphasia Therapy, pp. 97–134. University of Nebraska Medical Center, Omaha, 1977.

37. Luria, A. R.: Rehabilitation of Brain Functioning after War Traumas. Academy of Sciences Press, Moscow, 1948.
38. Luria, A. R.: Restoration of Function after Brain Injury. Macmillan, New York, 1963.
39. Luria, A. R.: Traumatic Aphasia: Its Syndromes, Psychology, and Treatment. Mouton, The Hague, 1970.
40. Luria, A. R.: The Man with a Shattered World. Basic Books, New York, 1972.
41. Marks, M., Taylor, M. L. & Rusk, H.: Rehabilitation of the aphasic patient: a survey of three years experience in a rehabilitation setting. Neurol 7: 837, 1957.
42. Messerli, P., Tissot, A. & Rodriguez, J.: Recovery from aphasia: some factors of prognosis. In: Y. Lebrun & R. Hoops (eds.), Recovery in Aphasics—Neurolinguistics 4, pp. 124–135. Swets & Zeitlinger, B.V., Amsterdam, 1976.
43. Mills, C.: Treatment of aphasia by training. J Amer Med Assoc 43: 1940, 1904.
44. Moss, C.: Recovery with Aphasia: The Aftermath of My Stroke. University of Illinois Press, Illinois, 1972.
45. Prins, R., Snow, C. & Wagenaar, E.: Recovery from aphasia: spontaneous speech versus language comprehension. Brain Lang 6: 192, 1978.
46. Reinvang, I.: Sentence production in recovery from aphasia. In: Y. Lebrun & R. Hoops (eds.), Recovery in Aphasics—Neurolinguistics 4, pp. 171–188. Swets & Zeitlinger, B.V., Amsterdam, 1976.
47. Ritchie, D.: Stroke: A Study of Recovery. Doubleday, New York, 1961.
48. Rose, C., Boby, V. & Capildeo, R.: A retrospective survey of speech disorders following stroke, with particular reference to the value of speech therapy. In: Y. Lebrun & R. Hoops (eds.), Recovery in Aphasics—Neurolinguistics 4, pp. 189–197.Swets & Zeitlinger, B.V., Amsterdam, 1976.
49. Russell, W. R. & Espir, M. L. E.: Traumatic Aphasia. Oxford University Press, London, 1961.
50. Sands, E., Sarno, M. T. & Shankweiler, D.: Long-term assessment of language function in aphasia due to stroke. Arch Phys Med Rehab 50: 203, 1969.
51. Sarno, J. E. & Sarno, M. T.: Stroke: The Condition and the Patient. McGraw-Hill, New York, 1969, 2nd edition, 1979.
52. Sarno, M. T.: Method for multivariant analysis of aphasia based on studies of 235 patients in a rehabilitation setting. Arch Phys Med Rehab 49: 210, 1968.
53. Sarno, M. T.: The Functional Communication Profile: manual of directions. Institute of Rehabilitation Medicine, New York University Medical Center, New York, 1969.
54. Sarno, M. T.: The status of research in recovery from aphasia. In: Y. Lebrun & R. Hoops (eds.), Recovery in Aphasics—Neurolinguistics 4, pp. 13–30. Swets & Zeitlinger, B.V., Amsterdam, 1976.
55. Sarno, M. T. & Levita, E.: Natural course of recovery in severe aphasia. Arch Phys Med Rehab 52: 175, 1971.
56. Sarno, M. T. & Levita, E.: Recovery in treated aphasia during the first year post-stroke. Stroke 10: 663–670, 1979.
57. Sarno, M. T., Silverman, M. & Sands, E.: Speech therapy and language recovery in severe aphasia. J Speech Hear Res 13: 607, 1970.
58. Schuell, H.: Auditory impairment in aphasia: significance and retraining techniques. J Speech Hear Dis 18: 14, 1953.
59. Schuell, H., Jenkins, J. & Jimenez-Pabon, E.: Aphasia in Adults. Harper & Row, New York, 1964.
60. Simonson, J.: According to the Aphasic Adult. University of Texas Southwestern Medical School, Texas, 1971.

61. Smith, A.: Objective indices of severity of chronic aphasia in stroke patients. J Speech Hear Dis 26: 167, 1971.
62. Smith, A.: Diagnosis, Intelligence and Rehabilitation of Chronic Aphasics. University of Michigan, Department of Physical Medicine and Rehabilitation, Ann Arbor, 1972.
63. Spreen, O. & Benton, A.: Neurosensory Center Comprehensive Examination for Aphasia: manual of directions. University of Victoria, Neuropsychology Laboratory, Victoria, B.C., 1969.
64. Stryker, S.: Speech after Stroke: A Manual for the Speech Pathologist and the Family Member. Charles C. Thomas, Springfield, Ill., 1975.
65. Taylor, M. L.: Understanding Aphasia: A Guide for Family and Friends. institute of Rehabilitation Medicine, New York University Medical Center, New York, 1958.
66. Taylor, M.L.: Language therapy. In: H. Burr (ed.), The Aphasic Adult: Evaluation and Rehabilitation, pp. 139–160. Wayside Press, Charlotesville, Va., 1964.
67. Taylor, M. L.: A measurement of functional communication in aphasia. Arch Phys Med Rehab 46: 101, 1965.
68. Taylor, M. L. & Marks, M.: The basic 100 words. Aphasia Rehabilitation Manual and Workbook. Institute of Rehabilitation Medicine, New York University Medical Center, New York, 1955.
69. Taylor, M. L. & Marks, M.: Aphasia Rehabilitation Manual and Therapy Kit. Institute of Rehabilitation Medicine, New York University Medical Center, New York, 1959.
70. Teuber, H.: Effects of brain wounds implicating right or left hemisphere in man. In: V. Mountcastle (ed.), Interhemispheric Relations and Cerebral Dominance, pp. 131–157. Johns Hopkins Press, Baltimore, 1962.
71. Vignolo, L.: Evolution of aphasia and language rehabilitation: a retrospective exploratory study. Cortex 1: 344, 1964.
72. Weisenberg, T. & McBride, K.: Aphasia: A Clinical and Psychological Study. Hafner, New York, 1964. (First edition: Commonwealth Fund, 1935.)
73. Wepman, J.: Recovery from Aphasia. Ronald Press, New York, 1951.
74. Wint, G.: The Third Killer: Meditations on a Stoke. Abelard-Schuman, New York, 1967.
75. Wulf, H.: Aphasia: My World Alone. Wayne State University Press, Michigan, 1973.
76. Yarnell, P., Monroe, P. & Sobel, L.: Aphasia outcome in stroke: a clinical neuroradiological correlation. Stroke 7: 514, 1976.

Analyzing aphasic behavior

MARTHA TAYLOR SARNO

CLASSIFICATION

Traditionally, the analysis of aphasic behavior is based, for the most part, on the results of tests which sample various verbal behaviors (e.g. naming). The pattern of symptoms observed is then related to a preconceived classification scheme. In the majority of instances the aphasia clinician is satisfied with clinical impressions as the basis for classification (39). Clearly, the most useful kind of classification system would be descriptive and prescriptive, that is, it would provide categories for all possible aphasic disorders. Schuell et al. (61) held that a system of classification for aphasia must be based on comprehensive observations of large numbers of aphasic subjects over long periods of time. She felt that without longitudinal studies to determine which symptoms are transient, which are persistent and which are interrelated there could be no stable classification system.

Weisenberg and McBride (69) pointed out that "Nowhere in the aphasia literature is confusion more evident than in the classification of types of disorders. There are differentiations on anatomical, physiological, and psychological grounds and on various combinations of these. Physiological differentiations have been most numerous. They are difficult to interpret, for the terms 'motor', 'sensory', 'visual', 'auditory', and so forth, have often been used to connote aspects of complex psychical activity. The difficulties inherent in this use of the terms caused Head (32) to reject them absolutely."

The difficulty of comprehending the phenomena of language in dissolution is merely an extension of the general lack of understanding of the organization of normal language processes. To add to the complexity, we might consider the fact that it is likely that language is inextricably intertwined in its organization with all cognitive, perceptual and emotional functions. It is, therefore, not surprising that classification has traditionally been based upon anatomical or gross clinical phenomena. Virtually nothing is known about the physiology of language upon which classification might be based. Only recently the techniques of modern linguistics have been applied to the study of aphasia and might possibly serve as a basis for future classification. Indeed, classification should ideally be multidimensional, identifying pathology in anatomic, physiologic, linguistic and possibly cognitive terms.

Recently Kertesz and Phipps (40) as well as Benson and Geschwind (3) expressed the view that the majority of authors accept the need for accurate classification as a basis for research and treatment and though there are seemingly discordant classification systems, certain frequently occurring and rare classes of aphasia are agreed upon by most clinicians. As stated above, most clinicians are satisfied with their clinical impressions as a basis for classification rather than performance on certain tests. The majority of investigations seem to support the traditional classification of aphasias.

In a recent paper by Brust et al. (11) he stressed that basing the study of an aphasia population on any classification is unlikely to produce new insights into whether the system being utilized accurately detects the physiological or psychological similarities or differences within the population. And as Spreen (64) points out "the nosological system chosen determines the scope and amount of detail available". Again, methodology dictates the facts. No scheme, therefore, is likely to produce more than a confirmation or lack of confirmation for the classification system used by the investigator. We cannot gain new insights into the usefulness of the nosological scheme employed or into the possibility of new types of syndromes of aphasia. This is why large scale research is often disappointing in its results if one expects more than epidemiologic statistics.

Brust adds, with deference to the existing classifications of aphasia, that it would be useful if we could find a more empirical way of confirming or altering our concepts of aphasic syndromes. At the moment we appear to have arrived at an almost hopeless impasse. The situation is not unlike that which exists in the classification of psychiatric disorders, where schemes of classification are related to either anatomical or psychological approaches.

Historically, many classifications of aphasia have been proposed and are based primarily on anatomical or psychological considerations. Benton's historical review (4) noted that virtually all of the currently recognized symptoms of aphasia had been described long before the nineteenth century. Jackson (37) classified aphasia according to psychological phenomena and rejected the idea that "pure" aphasia could be linked to specific areas of damage. Jackson's student, Henry Head (32) defined aphasia as "a disturbance of symbolic formulation and expression" and classified it as follows:

1. "*Verbal aphasia* consists of a difficulty in forming words for external or internal speech." The patient's ability to comprehend spoken or written content is usually considerably greater than is his ability for utterance or writing. "The disorder affects mainly verbal structure and words as integral parts of a phrase; their nominal value and significance remain relatively intact."

2. "*Syntactical aphasia* is essentially a disorder of balance and rhythm; syntax suffers greatly ... the patient has plenty of words, but their arrangement into coordinated phrases is defective ... Comprehension of the meaning of words, however, is always in excess of power to employ them in discourse."

3. "*Nominal aphasia* comprises loss of power to use names and want of comprehension of the significant value of words and other symbols ...

patients read with extreme difficulty, writing is grossly affected, and they suffer from defective appreciation of single numbers or letters."

4. "*Semantic aphasia* consists in a want of recognition of the full significance of words and phrases apart from their direct verbal meaning ... the patient may understand a word or a short phrase, but its ultimate significance escapes him and he fails to comprehend the final intention of some command imposed on him orally or in print."

Weisenberg and McBride

The classification scheme of Weisenberg and McBride (69) which was made more popular by Eisenson's (21) adoption of their system for his test *Examing for Aphasia* (21) classified patients into four general categories:

Predominantly Receptive: greatest disturbance in ability to comprehend spoken or written symbols.

Predominantly Expressive: greatest disturbance in ability to express ideas in speeech or writing.

Amnesic: chief difficulty in evocation of appropriate words.

Expressive-Receptive: both expressive and receptive extremely disturbed.

Goldstein

Goldstein believed that aphasic patient's deficits in abstracting, initiating and shifting behaviors, and grouping common properties and understanding whole concepts affected the overall reactions. He felt that the impairment in abstract attitude combined with personality changes affected the way in which aphasics handled verbal material and that all of the behaviors one observed in aphasic patients were manifestations of the organism's attempt to adjust to an altered condition. Goldstein (25) recognized several types of aphasia:

Expressive: peripheral motor, preserved writing, central motor (Broca's Aphasia), and transcortical motor (preserved repetition).

Receptive: pure word deafness, cortical sensory (Wernicke's Aphasia), and transcortical sensory.

Central Aphasia: (Wernicke's Conduction Aphasia).

Amnesic: (Word finding difficulty).

Wepman

Wepman (70) saw disturbances in aphasia as modality bound input and output deficits in direct contrast to Schuell's view that aphasia is a general language defect which crosses all language modalities. Wepman's classification and nomenclature follows:

Syntactic Aphasia: a disorder of symbol formulation in which the patient is unable to make use of previous knowledge of grammatical structure. Patients in this category tend to misuse or omit function words, speak telegraphically, and do not employ the normal stress and intonation characteristic of normal language use. They may retain many substantive words (nouns, verbs, adjectives) and often retain certain automatic phrases like "I don't know".

Semantic Aphasia: a disorder of symbol formulation in which the patient has difficulty recalling or using the meaningful verbal sign for a concept. These patients have difficulty remembering and using nouns, verbs, and adjectives except those which have the highest frequency of usage. They often circumlocute or use body or vocal gestures for expression.

Pragmatic Aphasia: a disorder of comprehension in which the patient has difficulty associating incoming signals with the appropriate concepts. Patients in this category are not usually aware of their errors. They generally retain the melody and pitch variations of normal speech and do not deviate appreciably from normal with respect to relative frequency of usage of the various parts of speech.

Jargon Aphasia: patients in this category use unintelligible sequences of phonemes, usually retaining the stress patterns of the language so that at times speech production sounds normal.

Global Aphasia: a degree of impairment in which the patient shows little or no ability to communicate in any modality. Global aphasics may perseverate, repeat meaningful phrases, or communicate to some degree through gesture and facial expression. If comprehension exists at all, it is generally limited to the patients immediate concerns. These patients often rely on primitive gesture and facial expression to express themselves. They often produce a meaningless repetition of sound combinations produced with intonation so that it appears that meaning is intended.

Schuell

Hildred Schuell arrived at a classification system on the basis of data obtained on her test, the *Minnesota Test for the Differential Diagnosis of Aphasia* (MTDDA) (60). She classified patients into five major categories as follows:

Group 1

Simple Aphasia: a reduction of available language in all modalities with no specific sensorimotor or perceptual impairment or dysarthria. These patients generally manifest word finding difficulties and reduced verbal retention span. Speech and writing are generally more impaired than auditory comprehension and reading. Patients in Group 1 tend to be younger, have little or no involvement of the extremities, and the lowest incidence in her patient sample of visual field defects, hypertension, emotional lability or other neurological impairments.

Group 2

Aphasia with Visual Involvement: reduction of available language in all modalities, with coexisting impairment of discrimination, recognition and recall of learned visual symbols. These patients may confuse letters with similar visual paterns or distort letters in writing. In this group, reading and writing are generally more impaired than speaking or auditory comprehension and there is a high incidence of visual field defects.

Group 3

Aphasia with Sensorimotor Involvement: severe reduction of language in all modalities accompanied by difficulty in discriminating, sequencing, and producing phonemes. Speech is generally telegraphic in style. Copying, drawing, and matching are usually not affected. Oral output is often slow and labored and the incidence of hemiplegia is high.

Group 4

Aphasia with Scattered Findings Compatible with Generalized Brain Damage: reduction of available language with scattered findings usually include both visual involvement and some dysarthria. There may be impairments in visual discrimination and spatial perception. Patients in this group are usually able to communicate functionally but with limitations.

Patients in Groups 4 and 5 tend to be older than those in other groups and have a high incidence of hypertension, previous strokes, organic mental deficits and cranial nerve pathology.

Group 5

Irreversible Aphasia Syndrome: this group is characterized by an almost complete loss of functional language skills in all modalities. Although these patients may be able to match pictures and words to pictures, they usually cannot name or point to objects, write or read single words or follow simple directions. They sometimes retain serial and automatic speech and everyday greetings, but functional propositional speech is essentially absent.

Luria

The noted Russian neuropsychologist, Alexander Luria (46, 47) designed a classification system derived from a Pavlovian model as follows:

Sensory Aphasia: a disturbance in the understanding of speech with defects in repetition, naming, writing, and spontaneous speech.

Acoustic Amnesic Aphasia: poor repetition when the amount of information the patient is required to process is increased

Afferent (Kinesthetic) Motor Aphasia: inability to make the oral movements fundamental to the production of phonemes which is reflected in defective pronunciation.

Efferent (Kinetic) Motor Aphasia: difficulty with the transition from sounds to phrases.

Semantic Aphasia: confusions of meaning, misunderstanding of spoken language.

Dynamic Aphasia: patient unable to propositionalize or express himself independently. No spontaneous speech.

The Mayo Clinic Group

Although it doesn't represent an independent classification system it is worth noting that the group at the Mayo Clinic (14) consider defects in aphasia which are primarily phonemic as representative of a separate aphasic syndrome which they call apraxia of speech (speech dyspraxia, verbal apraxia).

The following symptoms characterize the disorder:

1. Phonemic errors prominent (omissions, substitutions, distortions, additions, repetitions).
2. Some perseverative errors, others anticipatory.
3. Errors are approximations of desired production.
4. Errors are highly inconsistent.
5. Errors vary with complexity of articulatory adjustment.
6. Errors increase as words increase in length.
7. Discrepancy between articulatory accuracy displayed in automatic-reactive speech and the inaccuracy displayed in volitional-purposive performances.
8. Imitative responses are poor.
9. Speaker usually aware of his errors, but unable to anticipate or correct them.
10. Monitoring in anticipation of errors leads to prosodic disturbances such as slowed rate, even stress, even spacing.
11. Oral apraxia often, not always, observed in association with apraxia of speech.

Table I. *Aphasia classification by syndromes*
Geschwind (1971)

Type of aphasia	Site of lesion	Spontaneous speech	Compre-hension	Repeti-tion	Naming
Broca's aphasia	Posterior-inferior frontal	Non-fluent	Intact	Limited	Limited
Wernicke's aphasia	Posterior-superior temporal	Fluent	Impaired	Impaired	Impaired
Conduction aphasia	Arcuate-fasciculus	Fluent	Intact	Impaired	Impaired
Isolation syndrome	Association cortex	Fluent, echolalic	Impaired	Intact	Impaired
Anomic aphasia	Angular gyrus	Fluent	Intact	Intact	Impaired

The Boston School

Geschwind and his group at the Boston Veteran's Administration Hospital have adopted a classical anatomical approach to the classification of aphasia and have added the dimension of "fluency" as a factor of classification (3).

According to the "Boston School", the major subdivision among aphasic syndromes is based on the quality of spontaneous speech production, and can be correlated with the anatomical locus of the lesion (36).

According to these workers, analysis of the typology of aphasia from the classic writings of Broca and Wernicke to the present time reveals that the most significant difference between the major groups of patients resides in the character of their production, and not, as commonly assumed, in the opposition between the functions of language intake and language output (30). These workers believe that the notion of input and output as the major dimensions for classifying aphasic language disorders led to investigations using large scale analyses of test results; attention was directed away from differences in the pattern of *productive speech defects*, thought by them to be the most significant differentiating clue among the several types of aphasia (30).

An objective index of length of uninterrupted word-sequences was found to produce a sharp dichotomy in the aphasic population, separating Broca's aphasics from Wernicke and amnesic aphasics. This objective measure was reliably reproduced by several rating scales, including one which explicitly required a judgement as to the longest number of uninterrupted words in nonstereotyped sequences (30). Phrase/length ratio was found, on objective measurement, to be the basis for a sharp dichotomy in the aphasic population. This variable was conceived to reflect fluency of motor speech

Table II. *Classification systems*

Boston	Head	Gold-stein	Weisenberg & McBride	Luria	Wepman
Anomia	Nominal aphasia	Amnestic aphasia	Amnestic aphasia	Acoustic amnestic aphasia	Semantic aphasia
Wernicke's aphasia	Syntactic aphasia	Sensory aphasia	Predominantly receptive aphasia	Acoustic aphasia	Pragmatic aphasia
Broca's aphasia	Verbal aphasia	Motor aphasia	Predominantly expressive aphasia	Efferent motor aphasia	Syntactic aphasia
Conduction aphasia		Central aphasia		Afferent motor aphasia	
			Expressive-receptive aphasia		
Transcortical sensory aphasia (isolated speech area syndrome)					
Transcortical motor aphasia				Dynamic aphasia	

sequences. Goodglass et al. (30) concluded that by defining more precisely what to listen for, one could progress in identifying what is of paramount significance to the clinical classification of aphasia.

Table I outlines the syndromes of aphasia as viewed by the Boston group. The system has been widely accepted and currently forms the basis for most clinical studies.

Kerschensteiner et al. (38) attempted to investigate the reality of the fluency/non-fluency dichotomy and confirmed by statistical analysis that two distinct groups corresponding to the clinical syndromes of fluent and non-fluent aphasia did exist. The authors warned, however, of the dangers inherent in referring to aphasic patients as "posterior" or "anterior" aphasics, acknowledging the intimate association of anatomical facts but emphasizing that the fluent/non-fluent dichotomy is a behavioral-linguistic classification and is useful as such.

Wagenaar, Snow and Prins (68) using the variables of speech tempo and mean length of utterance also supported the concept of fluency as the basis for classifying aphasics. In this context, one should mention Brust's statement that it is not always easy to classify speech as fluent or non-fluent (11).

Conduction Aphasia has been the focus of considerable interest. Goldstein (24), Luria (47) and Brown (10) considered it a rare condition. Geschwind (personal communication, 1978) reports that 20% of all new admissions at the Boston Veteran's Administration Hospital are classified as conduction aphasics. In the Brust (11) review of 177 aphasic patients, 6% manifested conduction aphasic syndromes in the acute stroke stage. In my experience with an aphasic population more typical of the rehabilitation medicine setting, conduction aphasia is extremely rare.

Anatomical assumptions about the relationship of conduction aphasia to specific anatomical lesions (10, 11) remain open to debate. The repetition deficit seen in conduction aphasia was studied by Strub and Gardner (65) who concluded that it is a linguistic deficit associated specifically with the processing of sentences and ordering of phonemes.

Table II attempts to illustrate "equivalent" aphasic types according to the nomenclature used by different investigators.

As a summary statement of this section on classification one might say that if the purpose of nosology is to improve therapeutic efficiency we have not advanced substantially beyond the level of our nineteenth century colleagues. We are still in the descriptive stage since, beyond a loose correlation with an anatomical locus, fluency or non-fluency, give us neither a clue as to underlying pathophysiology nor any convincing guide on how to proceed therapeutically. Nevertheless, as with all scientific endeavors, this is a necessary early stage.

TESTS OF APHASIA

It is a general practice for the clinician engaged in the management of aphasic patients to administer a formal aphasia test to patients who demonstrate communication dysfunction secondary to brain damage.

Benton (5) and others interested in aphasia testing have made analogies between intelligence and aphasia testing on the grounds that first both intelligence and language are frequently impaired either in combination or separately, in adults with acquired cerebral disease and that the potential development of both intelligence and language, as well as their actual level of function at any given time, are strictly determined by central nervous system factors. Benton considers that the stage of aphasia testing is today where intelligence testing was in the 1900's, i.e. in the pre-Binet stage.

Many tests have been devised and used ... some have enjoyed wide use (such as the battery developed by Hildred Schuell) ... but no test or combination of tests has been so widely adopted as to make it generally recognized as "the" standard test for aphasia ... as Benton pointed out (5) ... none of the existing batteries could accomplish what the Binet or Wechsler scales have accomplished in the field of intellectual testing. He felt an important need for establishing something close to a standard examination in aphasia would go far towards establishing a level of *operational* understanding among workers ... a prerequisite for scientific communication in the field of aphasia.

In a psycholinguistic analysis of some frequently used aphasia tests, Osgood and Miron (49) emphasized the obvious redundancy in the test items encountered in available tests, and the fact that tests designed for the evaluation of specific dysfunctions must run the gamut of the various aspects of cognitive functions, as well as those functions of a more strictly motor and sensory nature.

Miron pointed out that tests which evolve from a strictly empirical frame of reference may fail to include items which might be suggested by a theoretical model, items which may well be highly significant from a diagnostic point of view. Thus, in general, a theoretical model generates predictions which may be submitted to empirical verification.

In the published proceedings of a conference on Aphasia held in Boston in 1958, Eisenson pointed out that in aphasia testing we are testing for factors correlated with the disorder rather than the entity itself. He questioned the need for extensive breadth and intensive depth in aphasia testing, particularly if the interest is primarily in rehabilitation. He also stressed the limits on objectivity in scoring as a consequence of the large number of variables operating in the determination of a patient's production or failure to produce a correct response at any particular moment. He did not want his test to result in a label for each patient, but rather a means to gain some insight into the patient's difficulties. Once the area of difficulty has been identified, more specialized tests can be used to obtain detailed information (49).

The following will briefly review some current widely used tests with particular reference to their uniqueness in method and assessment in the oral–aural (speech and comprehension) modalities.

Wepman and Jones (70) developed a differential psycholinguistic method in their *Language Modalities Test for Aphasia* for scoring responses according to input modality. The Visual test stimuli are contained on film strips and the examiner's voice presents auditory stimuli. The patient is required to give a narrative in spontaneous speech based on a picture depicting an activity. A 6 point scale for scoring oral and graphic responses instead of a pass/fail system is employed.

Errors are classified as:

a. Correct response.
b. Phonemic errors.
c. Grammatical and syntactic errors.
d. Semantic errors.
e. Jargon errors.
f. No response, admission of inability to respond or any automatic phrase.

An added feature is an 8 level, self-correction and recovery scale considered a prognostic indicator of a patient's language ability.

Hildred Schuell's (60) *Minnesota Test for Differential Diagnosis of Aphasia* (MTDDA) provides an in depth evaluation of five major areas:

a. Auditory disturbances (9 subtests): word recognition, sentence and paragraph comprehension.
b. Visual and reading disturbances (9 subtests): form matching, sentence/paragraph reading.
c. Speech and language disturbances (15 subtests): articulatory movement, naming, word definition, picture description.
d. Visuo-Motor and writing (10 subtests): copying, writing to dictation.
e. Numerical relations and arithmetic processes (4 subtests): clock setting, simple arithmetic, problem solving.

Each subtest contains items that vary in degree of complexity.

A 6 point clinical rating scale, ranging from no impairment to total impairment is provided for evaluating auditory, speech, reading and writing areas.

A *structured conversation* in which the patient is asked "What does your job involve?" and a *narrative* in which the patient is asked to tell a story describing a picture comprise the spontaneous speech sample on this test.

The Porch Index of Communicative Ability (PICA) (53) surveys lingusitic impairment using ten common objects as auditory, visual and tactile stimuli to elicit verbal, gestural, or graphic responses.

There is provision in this test for the derivation of an overall score, which is an average of all the means of the subtest means. It is considered the best single index of the patient's general communicative ability. It places the patient's performance on the test battery at a particular point on a sixteen step scale of adequacy, with 1.00 being the least adequate performance and 16.00 being the most adequate.

The scale indicates the accuracy, completeness, facility, promptness and responsiveness of a patient's reactions.

The shortcomings of the PICA include the fact that because of the multidimensional evaluation method, examiners must be "retrained" periodically in order to maintain inter-examiner reliability.

Also, determinations of such aspects of language as fluency and assessment of spontaneous speech are less than optimal and the range of stimuli is restricted (39).

The *Neurosensory Center Comprehensive Examination for Aphasia* (NCCEA) (65) consists of 20 tests of language performance and four control tests of visual and tactile functions (to detect the presence of visual or tactile deficits that might affect performance on language items). The test battery includes *Visual Naming, Word Fluency, Sentence Repetition* and the *Token Test.* Digits Forward and in Reverse as well as a test of *Sentence Construction* are also included.

The *Visual Naming* task requires that the patient name various common objects on visual confrontation (ie., cup). *Word Fluency* asks that the patient say as many words beginning with a specified letter as possible within one minute. *Sentence Repetition* requires the patient to repeat sentences of increasing length and grammatical complexity. The *Token Test* consists of 39 verbal commands of increasing complexity in which the patient manipulates twenty plastic tokens of two shapes, two sizes, and five colors. "Show me a circle" is an example of one of the simplest commands. "Put the white square behind the yellow circle" is one of the more difficult ones (16).

A distinctive feature of the NCCEA is the derivation of a profile of directly comparable percentile ranks available for both normals and aphasics.

Another aphasia test battery which is closely related in design and rationale to the NCCEA is the *Multilingual Aphasia Examination* (MAE) (5). This test, developed by a team of noted aphasiologists is intended as a measure which might provide uniformity of assessment in aphasia across language groups.

The *Boston Diagnostic Aphasia Examination* (BDAE) (29) is a comprehensive aphasia test which samples a wide range of complexity and covers many aspects of aphasic behavior. The test is standardized and contains 25 subtests. It also includes a severity rating scale and a profile of speech characteristics. Goodglass and Kaplan proposed three possible purposes for aphasia testing: "(1) diagnosis of presence and type of aphasic syndrome, leading to inferences concerning cerebral localization, (2) measurement of the level of performance over a wide range, for both initial determination and detection of change over time, and (3) comprehensive assessment of the assets and liabilities of the patient in all language areas as a guide to therapy". The Goodglass/Kaplan test provides Z score profiles for five major aphasic syndromes: Broca's aphasia, Wernicke's aphasia, anomic aphasia, conduction aphasia, and transcortical sensory aphasia. The scores obtained on this examination do not "automatically classify patients nor point to the optimum approach to therapy", as the authors acknowledge that the value of any aphasia test rests with the experience and skill of the examiner.

The primary areas which are assessed on the BDAE are:

1. Conversational and expository speech.
2. Auditory comprehension.
   a. Word discrimination.
   b. Body part identification.
   c. Complex ideational material.
3. Oral expression.
   a. Oral agility (i.e., pursing lips, rapid word repetition).
   b. Automatic speech (i.e., recitation of days of the week).
   c. Reciting, singing, rhythm.
   d. Word repetition.
   e. Phrase repetition.
   f. Word reading.

      g. Responsive naming.

      h. Visual confrontation naming.

      j. Body-part naming

      k. Animal-naming.

      l. Oral sentence-reading.

4. Understanding Written Language.

      a. Symbol and word discrimination.

      b. Phonetic association (Word recognition) (Comprehension of oral spelling).

      c. Word-picture making.

      d. Reading sentences and paragraphs.

5. Writing.

      a. Mechanics of writing.

      b. Recall of written symbols.

      c. Written Word-finding.

      d. Written formulation.

Two scales which rate the severity and quality of speech include the *Profile of Speech Characteristics* which allows for ratings based on a conversational and expository speech interview of six features of speech, namely: melody (intonation pattern); articulatory agility; grammatical form (variety); frequency of paraphasia; word finding (informational content in relation to fluency); and auditory comprehension.

The *Aphasia Severity Rating Scale* is a scale of capacity for oral communication ranging from "0" for "no communication possible" to "5" for "no perceptible handicap".

Speech production which is used as the basis for ratings of the quality and severity of speech are the 10 minute open-end conversation at the beginning of the test and the patient's descriptive narrative of a cookie theft picture.

The *Western Aphasia Battery* (WAB) (41) is essentially a modified version of the BDAE. On this battery, spontaneous speech is measured in terms of fluency and information content. A scale from 1 to 10 (–0– meaningless utterances to –10– normal fluency) is included. Ratings are derived from responses to standardized conversational question and a picture description.

THE ANALYSIS OF SPONTANEOUS SPEECH

Spontaneous speech is a feature of language which is not readily reducible to objective measurement. It does not lend itself to "pass-fail" or numerical scoring ... yet it is the behavioral area which most reflects *aphasia*. Speech is a distinctive, unique behavior, markedly individual, intimately related to personality, cultural, and social-educational factors. As Prins emphasized, "... it (speech) is without doubt the skill in which improvement is most vital to the patient–and it is the area in which the patient feels his loss most" (54).

A number of studies have made detailed analyses of speech under conditions of open-ended conversation and/or free narrative for the purpose of attempting to specify the linguistic nature of aphasic deficits, in particular, the syndromes of aphasia (22, 23, 28, 43, 62, 71).

As mentioned earlier, there has also been research interest in establishing the basis for traditional as well as more contemporary views of classification through analyses of spontaneous speech in narration and conversation (2, 3, 68).

What is striking in the aphasia literature, however, is the virtual absence of procedures using spontaneous speech as a basis for conclusions and refinements about aphasia and a practical method for the analysis of spontaneous speech behavior in the clinical, as opposed to the research setting.

The potential knowledge which could be acquired from the application of purely linguistic criteria to the careful analysis of spontaneous speech in aphasia has been suggested.

Apart from some work of Lebrun (43), Reinvang (56) and Ludlow (45) few have used the technique of tape recording and transcribing a speech corpus as a research method.

Using a traditional philology method, three British linguists (57) provided a phonetic transcription of two tape recorded interviews with an aphasic patient. They suggested the need for studying a corpus of texts from acutely dysphasic patients, a view supported by Dr Critchley.

Wagenaar, Snow and Prins (68) in Amsterdam, mention their views of several deficiencies inherent in published analyses of spontaneous speech in aphasia:

1. The items are scored in a subjective and nonquantified manner which makes replication or application of the same scales to other samples impossible.
2. The analyses do not attempt a characterization of the grammatical structure in the produced speech.
3. The situation in which the spontaneous speech is elicited is too variable from patient to patient to allow strict comparison. In general, no information is even offered concerning the analyzed speech samples, where and how they were collected, what the topic was, etc. Yet it is known that variables such as the speech situation (informal vs. formal context), picture description vs. free narrative, the emotional state of the patient or the topic discussed can greatly influence the amount and character of the speech output of aphasic patients.

Based on the premise that spontaneous speech is important because it provides the most subtle and complete reflection of language abilities, especially if it can be analyzed in sufficient detail and subjected to adequate linguistic interpretation, Wagenaar and his colleagues devised a linguistic scheme which, in its modified form, seems to be quite practical.

The scheme for analyzing a tape recording of speech sample consists of 28 variables (i.e., tempo of speech, mean length of utterance, neologisms, etc.) which are counted or calculated in a variety of pre-specified ways (i.e., for tempo of speech: number of words produced in 6 minutes; for neologisms: number of neologisms expressed as percentage of number of content words). (See Table III.)

The Amsterdam group has designed a splendid method for quantifying the spontaneous speech of aphasics. One of the problems, of course that these workers had to confront was the decision concerning which segment of speech should be considered a reasonable unit for calculation. They decided that segmentation would be done according to the rule that syntactic criteria would be primary, melodic criteria secondary, and the presence of pauses least important.

In addition to calculating the 28 spontaneous speech variables, the scheme allows for counting the number of seconds of speech which are phonologically, syntactically, or semantically incomprehensible on a time basis. Repetitions of the examiner's utterances are counted as a measure of the inability to use language creatively or independently as are automatisms and self-corrections.

In addition to the 28 spontaneous speech variables their technique includes a severity scale which they call the *Communicative Capacity Index*, much like the scale of Goodglass and Kaplan (28). Patients who could say nothing that made sense received 1 while a score of 7 was given to someone indistinguishable from normal in terms of amount and precision of information. The intervening points for scores were defined precisely, e.g., patients who communicated inadequately, partly because they reacted inappropriately to questions and comments, partly because what little they did say was deficient in content and structure received a score of 3.

From the aphasia clinician's point of view the measurement of spontaneous speech in aphasia seems to be a dimension of aphasic behavior which we have tended to avoid and neglect. Since few concrete and practical schemes for quantifying spontaneous speech are provided by most published aphasia tests we have been satisfied to describe what the patient's speech sounds like, using terms which do not represent standard nomenclature.

Granting that the measurement of spontaneous speech in aphasia is fraught with seemingly insurmountable problems, there are, nonetheless, some methods, traditionally and particularly associated with linguistics, which have potential, practical application (68).

Until we attempt to objectify our patient's spontaneous speech behavior in everyday practice we will not have adequate, replicable means for assessing recovery and rehabilitation; evaluating with any objectivity the fluency/non-fluency dimension of speech behavior; and designing adequate treatment programs.

Table III. *Thirty variables selected for factor analysis*

Wagenaar, Snow, Prins (1975)

Variable	Method of calculation
Speech tempo	Number of words produced in 6 min
Communicative capacity	Average of the evaluations of each 2 min sample
Syntactic complexity	Average of the evaluation of each utterance
Melody	Average of the evaluations of each 2 min sample
Articulation	Average of the evaluations of each 2 min sample
Utterance production	Number of utterances produced in 6 min
Utterances shorter than five words	Number of utterances shorter than five words expressed as percentage of total number of utterances
Mean length of utterance	Number of words divided by number of utterances
Mean length of three longest utterances	Number of words in three longest utterances divided by 3
Complex utterances	Number of complex utterances expressed as percentage of total number of utterances
Seconds incomprehensible	Number of seconds of speech which were incomprehensible in 6 min
Self corrections	Number of self corrections expressed as percentage of total number of utterances
Automaticisms	Number of automatisms expressed as percentage of total number of utterances
Imitations	Number of imitations of the test assistant expressed as percentage of total number of utterances
Literal paraphasias	Number of literal paraphasias expressed as percentage of number of content words
Verbal paraphasias	Number of verbal paraphasias expressed as percentage of number of content words
Neologisms	Number of neologisms expressed as percentage of number of content words
Literal perseverations	Number of literal perseverations expressed as percentage of number of utterances
Verbal perseverations	Number of verbal perseverations expressed as percentage of number of utterances
Function-word substitutions	Number of substitutions of function words expressed as percentage of number of function words
Function-word deletions	Number of deletions of function words expressed as percentage of number of utterances
Content-word deletions	Number of deletions of content words expressed as percentage of number of utterances
Syntactic mixtures	Number of syntactically confused structures expressed as percentage of number of utterances
Content-word function-word ratio	Ratio of number of content words to number of function words
Nouns	Number of nouns expressed as percentage of total number of words
Personal pronouns	Ration of all pronouns to number of content words
Word-order mistakes	Number of word-order mistakes expressed as percentage of number of utterances
Tense mistakes	Number of tense mistakes expressed as percentage of number of utterances
Unclassified mistakes	Number of all other kinds of grammatical mistakes expressed as percentage of number of utterances

COMMENTS ON THE MEASUREMENT
OF AUDITORY COMPREHENSION

An excellent review of the history of thought concerning the measurement of comprehension in aphasia is contained in a recent paper by Boller (8). He emphasizes how little attention has been paid to this aspect of aphasic behavior, and how this is probably due to the fact that the receptive component is, at times, less striking than the verbal output deficit. Also, that "the analysis of comprehension can be based only on patient's responses to external stimuli, and these responses may be confounded by expressive disorders".

The notion that there are varieties of auditory comprehension deficits which are not necessarily sensitive to existing tests and measurements is not new. Clinicians are acutely aware of the inconsistencies and discrepancies exhibited by many aphasic patients for what seem to be differentially impaired aspects, or dimensions, of the behavior inclusive under the global term: Auditory Comprehension.

By the same token, clinicians and investigators have been frustrated by the many technical difficulties inherent in obtaining behavioral measures of comprehension. For example, isolating auditory comprehension from intellectual function and determining which failures on tasks of auditory comprehension are due to a "decoding" deficit and which are associated with difficulty in grasping the idea, (the concept) of a message is virtually imposible (16). DeRenzi and Vignolo (16) list the following qualities of a good test of auditory comprehension:

1. It should require a short period ot time for administration.
2. It should require neither special apparatus nor specific printed material (Pierre Marie's *Paper Test* was particularly suited to meet this requirement!).
3. It should be made up of orders so short as to be easily memorized by any normal adult regardless of age.
4. It should include the least possible difficulty on an intellectual level, so that any individual may be able to perform the tasks correctly, independently within reasonable limits—of his intellectual level of function.
5. It should contain, on the contrary, considerable difficulties on a linguistic level.

With respect to the meaning of the designation "difficulties on a linguistic level" the authors explain that the difficulties must lie on the lack of redundancy of the message transmitted to the patient and in the necessity, which this entails, of grasping its significance from the semantic value of every single word he hears. Lack of redundancy to this extent rarely occurs in every day conversation ... since the normal comprehension of speech is aided by many linguistic and some extralinguistic factors which contribute towards orienting the expectation set of the listener to a given direction, so that he merely needs to understand some of the elements of the message in order to respond appropriately. These extra clues include: the situation itself (speech during a medical exam); the verbal context of the message (the fact that the object talked about is there or not); etc.

TEMPORAL FACTORS

In an effort to further understand the nature of the auditory comprehension deficits observed in aphasia, some investigators have studied the temporal factors which might affect an individual patient's level of comprehension. This is probably related to the notion presented by Lenneberg (44) that "aphasia can be viewed as difficulty in temporal sequencing".

Efron (20) considered that aphasia might be primarily a defect in "temporal analysis" ... in placing a 'time-label' on incoming (data) material. He manipulated paired pure tones in a study of this variable and reported that aphasics required longer time intervals between sounds to sequence them correctly.

Ebbin and Edwards (19) manipulated real speech sounds, specifically syllables (in contrast to pure tones) and found that aphasics made significantly more errors than control patients when silent periods between syllables were short rather than long. This finding was also related to level of auditory comprehension but was not related to auditory recognition or auditory retention.

In a study of a patient with word deafness the understanding of spoken language improved dramatically when the examiner spoke at an abnormally slow rate. This rate-dependent linguistic processing defect was limited to the auditory modality (1).

In another study in which speech was introduced at normal, expanded (30 and 50%) and compressed (30 and 50%) rates, groups of aphasics showed greater impairment in listening to compressed speech than expanded speech (which is inconsistent with the clinical practice of speaking at a slower than normal rate when interacting with aphasic patients). "It is possible that general listening habits may be so dependent upon normal speaking rates that any severe deviation from these rates may have a detrimental effect." In general, this study did not support the notion that aphasic patients as a group respond significantly differently to compressed or expanded speech than normals (there was a difference noted between older age aphasics and normals, however) (17).

Parkhurst (51) compared responses of aphasic and non-aphasic subjects to spoken commands of varied length and complexity where the rate was manipulated by electronically compressing or expanding the speech signal by 35%. Aphasic subjects performed significantly more poorly in the compressed speech condition for all types of sentences. Some subjects improved in the expanded condition on longer, more difficult sentences.

ACOUSTIC VARIABLES

Blumstein et al. (7) investigated the voice onset time (VOT) dimension in aphasia to assess the ability of aphasics and non-aphasic brain damaged subjects to discriminate these stimuli and to relate this finding to type of aphasia and language comprehension skill. Voice onset time has been carefully investigated in normals and signals a phonetic dimension which is found in nearly all languages of the world. It would seem that if the phonetic and ultimately phonological form of words is incorrectly perceived, further analysis of auditory input in terms of semantic and syntactic attributes will be incorrect. However, in this study there was little correlation between patient's auditory language comprehension and ability to do speech perception tasks. In fact, one Wernicke's patient with the most severe comprehension deficit performed normally on the perception of VOT. The authors postulated that their findings supported the possibility that although a patient may be unable to perceive minimally redundant material he may nonetheless make use of all of the redundancies provided in natural language and consequently evidence moderately good auditory language comprehension. The results of this study lent support to the notion that Wernicke's patients have a greater comprehension deficit—this group of patients had difficulty assigning a stable category label to an auditory stimulus.

LEXICAL AND SYNTACTIC VARIABLES

Parisi and Pizzamiglio (50) pointed out that most tests of auditory comprehension evaluated the "global" effectiveness of language comprehension, and rarely specify the comprehension of specific syntactic rules ... in their study they found almost no differences between diagnostic groups with respect to comprehension of syntactically different material. Their data when compared with the results of groups of children 3 to 6 years of age showed the dissolution of syntactic comprehension in aphasia to highly correlate with the order of acquisition of the same rules in children.

Using the *Peabody Picture Vocabulary Test*, Goodglass et al., (27) studied breadth of vocabulary, auditory sequential pointing span, directional prepositions, and recognition of prepositions. When compared to normal adults and children, aphasics were vastly different in their ability to comprehend and showed patterns of auditory comprehension deficit which further validated the existence of distinctive diagnostic groups (i.e., Broca's, Wernicke's).

The effect of syntactic, vacabulary and sentence length on auditory comprehension was studied by Shewan and Canter (63) who found that different diagnostic groups definitely differed in their comprehension ability, with Wernicke's patients being the most impaired. Syntactic complexity, in their study, was the variable which was the most difficult parameter for all subjects.

In spite of the gross clinical differences with respect to comprehension in the various aphasic syndromes, Poeck, Kerschensteiner and Hartje (52) found equal impairment in auditory comprehension in both fluent and non-fluent aphasics. Parisi and Pizzamiglio (50) found no difference in the heirachy of difficulty of syntactic contrasts between Broca's and Wernicke's aphasics. It was the feeling of Prins, Snow and Wagenaar (54) that many studies which relied exclusively on the *Token Test* or on tests of a few morphological or syntactical rules might not exhaustively explore possible differences in comprehension deficits between subgroups of aphasics.

SEMANTIC FACTORS

Some processes of decoding seem preserved in even the most severe global aphasic. As Boller and Green (9) pointed out, some patients do not adequately respond to Yes/No questions, or point to objects on command, but may execute commands for whole body movements such as stand, turn, sit. Their study supported the idea that the process of decoding messages is not unitary but complex and that in some way even the most severe aphasic patients have an ability to make certain kinds of discriminations. They characteristically reject a foreign language and phonemic jargon as incomprehensible. These investigators believe that their inability to respond correctly to the messages they perceive is perhaps related to detailed semantic analyses being a separate and later stage of comprehension.

On the basis of a case study, Yamadori and Albert (72) suggested that perhaps the process of decoding meaning is independent in certain categories. Meaning categories such as body parts, room objects, or colors may have a more or less independent existence.

Needham and Swisher (48) systematically evaluated the relative difficulty of three tests of auditory comprehension and the effects of differences in test administration and scoring on test outcome. The tests were the *Token Test*; a structured language test (modeled after the MTDDA of Schuell); and the Understanding subcategory of the *Functional Communication Profile* (FCP), which is a clinical rating scale. The results of the study supported a clearcut difference in level of difficulty of the *Token Test* which revealed mild deficits most effectively but was limited in assessing the severely impaired patient because few responses could be elicited to the command, and, the FCP, which elicited responses from aphasics with difficulties throughout the range of impairment.

In his analysis of the grammar of aphasic patients, Goodglass (26) developed an interesting construct that perhaps sets the keynote for this section (characteristies of stimulus): the notion of *saliency*. Saliency was defined as "the psychologic resultant of the stress, the informational significance, the phonological prominence, and the affective value of a word". The data appear to indicate that the patient's comprehension of language and more especially the patient's fluency in initiating language depend upon the saliency of words; the patient apparently needs a salient word in order to initiate speech; when he is asked to repeat phrases, some opening with nonsalient function words and some with salient substantive words, he has more trouble initiating phrases with the former than with the latter. The implication is that in therapy we might help the patient initiate speech by making it easy for him to get hold of a salient word. Repetition is easier if sentences are constructed so as to allow a quick clutching of this salient word. Saliency appears to be a germinal notion which can help us think about several aspects of the stimulus (15).

Determining a patient's ability to understand speech remains one of the most difficult, yet essential, tasks faced by the clinician who evaluates aphasic patients. Performance clearly depends on several variables: temporal, acoustic, phonological, lexical, syntactical, semantic. In addition, some extra-linguistic factors seem to affect performance: the test situation, whether or not the topic at hand is of interest or familiar, the patient's level of fatigue, and the set or expectation.

At this time the clinician would probably fare best by using a systematic clinical rating of auditory comprehension derived from an informal conversation with the patient combined with the *Token Test* and one or two other tests which attempt to specifically assess the comprehension of independently lexical, syntactic, and semantic features. No combination of these, however, is a substitute for an imaginative clinician who spends long periods of time with the patient and begins to tune in to his particularly idiosyncratic decoding mechanisms.

COMMENTS ON FUNCTIONAL MEASUREMENT

Thirty years ago, Dr Edgar Doll (18), a psychologist, finding that I.Q. testing did not describe how patients used their mental capacities, developed the *Vineland Social Maturity Scale* as a measure of function in retardates. Actual behaviors (i.e., pulls off socks, eats with fork, cares for self at table, makes telephone calls) constituted the items rated on the scale since his concern was with all inclusive behaviors rather than elements which contributed to the performance of a particular behavior.

Yarnell et al. (73) stated that the families of the poor outcome patients often felt that their communication abilities were better than the low testing scores implied. This is probably an effect of environmental, gestural and other nonverbal cues used in familiar home situations. Thus the ratings of aphasia outcome must be considered relative at present.

Rationale for functional frame of reference in Aphasia

Experience in the field of rehabilitation medicine has shown that the level of physical function sometimes gives no clues as to the ability of a patient to function in life. This variation (discrepancy) is related to the interactive influence of physical, psychological, social, economic and cultural factors. Since practitioners of rehabilitation medicine have a particular interest in function, several rating scales have been designed to assess function. The most widely used functional scale is the *Activities of Daily Living* (ADL) (42) a scale which evaluates how much use a patient makes of residual muscle function to perform the tasks necessary for self care (feeding, dressing, toileting, etc.). Another scale, the *Functional Life Scale* (FLS) (59) was designed in a rehabilitation medicine setting for the purpose of rating how a patient is living at any given moment. This scale includes social, ADL, cognitive activities, and a composite of those areas which best reflect overall life function.

Most work in aphasia has generally focused on classification and phenomenology. This frame of reference probably accounts for why most aphasia tests emphasize finding deficits rather than describing residuals. The tests have concerned themselves with identifying "what" the patient said not "how" he communicates.

At a conference held in Boston in 1958, Dr Joe Brown stated that formal psychological testing is most useful for describing what an aphasic patient cannot do; it does not ordinarily tell us what he *does* in his attempts to circumvent his difficulties. A patient who may respond to none of the formal test comprehension items may respond appropriately when casually asked a question.

While analytic, in depth testing is fundamental to our understanding of aphasic deficits and as a basis for designing treatment and measuring progress, it is sometimes difficult to translate these findings into everyday terms (i.e., can the patient return to work, can he cope with his life situation). There appears to be a dimension of language performance which is not reflected in formal testing—a dimension of performance in natural language use, in contrast to performance which is sampled in artificial testing situations. Also, most of our evaluation techniques provide descriptions of patient capability during brief time intervals under relatively standardized conditions (31).

Uniqueness of the language user

In addition to the factors already mentioned which contribute to a need for evaluating natural language use, as opposed to responses to formal test items, there is a uniqueness about each language user which obliges us to take into account each individual's language world. "Each person's manner of using language is something individual and personal, which he never together shares with the rest of the community; it is something which reflects his total personality, in the same way as his handwriting or bodily mannerisms" (12, 13).

Approaches to functional measurement

A few measures have been designed which attempt to assess actual language use in aphasia. The *Functional Communication Profile* (FCP) (58, 67) consists of 45 behaviors considered common communication functions of everyday life, rated on a 9 point scale on the basis of informal interaction with the patient in a conversational situation.

Scores are obtained in Movement, Speech, Understanding, Reading and a Miscellaneous category which includes calculation and writing. Weighted scores are converted into percentages in each of the five modalities shown on the FCP form. The overall score reflects the sum of the weighted part scores and can be used as a single measure of an individual's communicative effectiveness in his everyday life.

On a Norwegian version of the FCP the number of scoring categories have been reduced from 8 to 4 and the items have been regrouped under 3 headings instead of the original 5.

The grouping of items on the Norwegian scale was based on factor analysis. The Norwegian functional groups are Primary Expressive abilities (attempt to communicate, ability to indicate yes and no, etc.; Primary Receptive abilities; and Secondary Linguistic skills (55).

Communication abilities of daily living (CADL) (33, 34, 35)

CADL designed by Audrey Holland (1976) attempts to incorporate both natural language activities and natural style in an effort to more closely approximate normal communication. CADL utilizes a 3-point scoring system: 0, 1, 2 (0 = wrong, 1 = adequate, 2 = correct). The scoring system allows for "close to correct" responses rather than the usual all or none, and this is desirable. Administration of the CADL is in the form of an interview with the examiner following a script. The interview begins with structured conversation such as "Do you have any children?" "How did your speech difficulty come about?" The next phase of the test involves role playing situations with props such as pretending to be in a doctor's office ("well, Mr/Ms ..., what has been bothering you lately?") or shopping (buying a notebook). It is difficult to assess natural language use under conditions which require an aphasic patient to pretend that he is in a real-life situation. While some of the items are especially good at simulating real life, others appear to rely on the comprehension of difficult directions and an intact ability to abstract. Nevertheless, the CADL is an example of an attempt to quantify natural language use in aphasia and as such represents a novel approach.

Summary

I have discussed some of the ways in which aphasia is classified, measured by tests, and my own views concerning measures of spontaneous speech and auditory comprehension, specifically those channels which utilize the speech code ... the code most vulnerable to aphasic deficits. Our methods of analysis remain primitive—we need to bear in mind some of the dimensions of the alterations in aphasia, and these require some imaginative assessment techniques.

Gardner (24) has said that although the brain-damaged individual remains in our society, he has suffered a blow that immediately places him on a new footing. Perhaps the least we should do is to meet him halfway, to determine which skills and aspects of symbolization remain, and to asess his competence in these latter areas ... if we want to ascertain his flexibility with objects, we should offer him not triangles and circles, but rather foods, or records, or friends, or other materials more likely to be evocative for his troubled mind.

He goes on to say that "A more instructive way to envision the world of the brain-damaged is to note the tremendous variation in a patient's performance from day to day. I have never seen a brain-damaged individual, with the possible exception of those either completely demented or virtually recovered, who did not display sizable variations in performance from day to day, if not across hours or minutes. This range is no mere outcome of chance: it is blatantly evident in the early stages of recovery and may be endemic to the condition of the braindamaged person. No skill seems to be completely destroyed or wholly intact; rather, each seems to be in a partial state of disrepair, and, depending upon such factors as the surrounding conditions, the extent of fatigue, the events of the preceding minutes, motivation at the given moment, the degree of alertness or attentiveness, the patient may succeed strikingly or fail dismally on a given set of tasks. This variability is all-important, because it precludes a ready, foolproof description of the patient—as most consulting physicians soon learn, one must speak of the patient at-a-given-moment-in-time, or in particular circumstances, rather than as a fixed set of mechanized routines, always performing at the same level."

Gardner has also emphasized that we cannot be sure to what extent patients would react to therapies and tests which are couched in relatively more familiar, personalized symbolic forms. As with any assessment of individuals from different cultures, the conclusions we draw about our aphasic patients must be regarded as highly tentative, inviting major revisions.

References

1. Albert, M. & Bear, D.: Time to understand: a case of word deafness with reference to the role of time in auditory comprehension. Brain 97: 373, 1957.
2. Benson, D.: Fluency in aphasia: correlation with radioactive scan localization. Cortex 8: 373, 1967.
3. Benson, D. & Geschwind, N.: The aphasias and related distrubances. In: H. B. Baker & L. H. Baker (eds.), Clinical Neurology. Vol. I. Harper & Row, New York, 1971.
4. Benton, A.: Contributions to aphasia before broca. Cortex 3: 32–58, 1964.
5. Benton, A.: Problems of test construction in the field of aphasia. Cortex 3: 32, 1967.
6. Benton, A.: Development of a multilingual aphasia battery: progress and problems. J Neurol Sci 9: 39, 1969.

7. Blumstein, S., Cooper, W., Zurif, E. & Caramazza, A.: Levels of speech perception dissociated in aphasia. Paper presented at Academy of Aphasia, October 1975.
8. Boller, F.: Comprehension disorders in aphasia: a historical review. Brain Long 5: 149, 1978.
9. Boller, F. & Green, E.: Comprehension in severe aphasics. Cortex 8: 382, 1972.
10. Brown, J. W.: Aphasia, Apraxia, Agnosia: Clinical and Theoretical Aspects. Charles C. Thomas, Springfield, Ill., 1972.
11. Brust, J., Shafer, S., Richter, R. & Bruun, B.: Aphasia and caute stroke. Stroke 7: 167, 1976.
12. Critchley, M.: Aphasiology and Other Aspects of Language. Edward Arnold Publications, London, 1970.
13. Critchley, M.: Artuculatory defects in aphasia. J Laryngol 66: 1–17, 1952.
14. Darley, F.: Nomenclature of expressive speech disturbances resulting from lesions in Broca's area: 108 years of proliferation and confusion. Paper presented at Academy of Aphasia, Boston, September 1969.
15. Darley, F.: A retrospective view: aphasia. J Speech Hear Dis 42: 161, 1977.
16. DeRenzi, E. & Vignolo, L.: The Token Test: a sensitive test to detect receptive disturbances in aphasia. Brain 85: 655, 1962.
17. DiCarlo, L. & Taub, H.: The influence of compression and expansion on the intelligibility of speech by young and aged aphasic (demonstrated CVA) individuals. J Comm Dis 5: 299, 1972.
18. Doll, E.: Vineland Social Maturity Scale: manual of directions. Educational Publishers, Philadelphia, 1947.
19. Ebbin, J. & Edwards, A.: Speech sound discrimination of aphasics when intersound interval is varied. J Speech Hear Res 10: 120, 1967.
20. Efron, F.: Temporal perception, aphasia and déjà vu. Brain 86: 403, 1963.
21. Eisenson, J.: Examining for Aphasia and Related Disturbances. Psychological Corporation, New York, 1954.
22. Fillenbaum, S., Jones, L. & Wepman, J.: Some linguistic features of speech from aphasic patients. Language Speech 4: 92, 1961.
23. Fry, D.: Phonemic substitutions in an aphasic patient. Language Speech 2: 52, 1959.
24. Gardner, H.: The Shattered Mind. Alfred Knopf, New York, 1975.
25. Goldstein, K.: Language and Language Disturbances. Grune & Stratton, New York, 1948.
26. Goodglass, H.: Studies on the grammar of aphasics. In H. Goodglass & S. Blumstein (eds.), Psycholinguistics and Aphasia, pp. 183–215. Johns Hopkins University Press, Baltimore, 1973.
27. Goodglass, H., Gleason, J. B., Berholtz, N. & Hyde, M.: Some linguistic structures in the speech of a Broca's aphasic. Cortex 8: 191, 1972.
28. Goodglass, H., Gleason, J. B. & Hyde, M.: Some dimensions of auditory language comprehension in aphasia. J Speech Hear Res 13: 595, 1970.
29. Goodglass, H. & Kaplan, E.: Boston Diagnostic Aphasia Examination. Lea & Febiger, Philadelphia, 1972.
30. Goodglass, H., Quadfasel, F. & Timberlake, W.: Phrase length and the type and severity of aphasia. Cortex 1: 133, 1964.
31. Halstead, L.: Longitudinal unobtrusive measurement in rehabilitation. Arch Phys Med Rehab 57: 189, 1976.
32. Head, H.: Aphasia and Kindred Disorders of Speech. Vols. I & II. Hafner, New York, 1963. (First edition: Cambridge University Press, 1926.)
33. Holland, A.: Communicative Adequacy of Daily Living. University of Pittsburgh, Pittsburgh, 1976.

34. Holland, A.: Estimators of aphasic patients' communicative performance in daily life. Final Report. National Institute of Neurology and Communicative Disorders and Stroke, Washington, D.C., 1977.
35. Holland, A.: Some practical considerations in aphasia rehabilitation. In: M. Sullivan & M. Krommers (eds.), Rationale for Adult Aphasia Therapy, pp. 167–180. University of Nebraska Medical Center, Omaha, 1977.
36. Howes, D. & Geschwind, N.: Quantitative studies of aphasic language. Ass Res Nerv Ment Dis 42: 229, 1964.
37. Jackson, H.: On the nature of the duality of the brain. Med Press & Circular 1, 19, 41, 65, 1864. (Reprinted in Brain 38: 80, 1915.)
38. Kerschensteiner, M., Poeck, K. & Brunner, E.: The fluency non-fluency dimension in the classification of aphasic speech. Cortex 8: 233, 1972.
39. Kertesz, A. & McCabe, P.: Recovery patterns and prognosis in aphasia. Brain 100, 1977.
40. Kertesz, A. & Phipps, J.: Numerical taxonomy of aphasia. Brain Lang 4: 1977.
41. Kertesz, A. & Poole, E.: The aphasia quotient: the taxonomic approach to measurement of aphasic disability. Canadian J Neurol Sci 1: 7–16, 1974.
42. Lawton, E.: Activities of Daily Living for Physical Rehabilitation. McGraw-Hill, New York, 1963.
43. Lebrun, Y.: Linguistic analysis of two cases of emissive aphasia. J Neurol Sci 4: 271, 1967.
44. Lenneberg, E.: Biological Foundations of Language. Wiley & Sons, New York, 1967.
45. Ludlow, C.: Recovery from aphasia: a foundation for treatment. In: M. Sullivan & M. Krommers (eds.), Rationale for Adult Aphasia Therapy, pp. 97–134. University of Nebraska Medical Center, Omaha, 1977.
46. Luria, A. R.: Factors and forms of aphasia. In: A. V. S. de Reuck & M.O' Connor (eds.), Disorders of Language, pp. 143–167. Little Brown, Boston, 1964.
47. Luria, A. R.: Human Brain and Psychological Processes. Harper & Row, New York, 1966.
48. Needham, L. S. & Swisher, L. P.: A comparison of three tests of auditory comprehension for adult aphasics. J Speech Hear Dis 37: 123, 1972.
49. Osgood, C. & Miron, M. Approaches to the Study of Aphasia. University of Illinois, Urbana, Ill., 1963.
50. Parisi, D. & Pizzamiglio, L.: Syntactic comprehension in aphasia. Cortex 6: 204, 1970.
51. Parkhurst, B.: The effect of time altered speech stimuli on the performance of right hemiplegic adult aphasics. Paper presented at the American Speech and Hearing Association Convention, New York, November, 1970.
52. Poeck, K., Kerschensteiner, M. & Hartje, W.: A quantitative study of language understanding in fluent and non-fluent aphasia. Cortex 8: 299, 1972.
53. Porch, B.: Porch Index of Communicative Ability. Vol. II. Administration, Scoring, and Interpretation. Consulting Psychologists Press, California, 1967.
54. Prins, R., Snow, C. & Wagenaar, E.: Recovery from aphasia: spontaneous speech versus language comprehension. Brain Lang 6: 192–211, 1978.
55. Reinvang, I.: Functional language in aphasia. Scnad J Rehab Med 1: 112, 1969.
56. Reinvang, I.: Sentence production in recovery from aphasia. In: Y. Lebrun & R. Hoops (eds.), Recovery in Aphasics—Neurolinguistics 4, pp. 171–188. Swets & Zeitlinger, B.V., Amsterdam, 1976.
57. Ross, A., Clarke, P. & Haddock, N.: Edition of text from a dysphasic patient. In: A. V. S. deReuck & M. O'Connor (eds.), Disorders of Language, pp. 299–317. Little Brown, Boston, 1964.

58. Sarno, M. T.: The Functional Communication Profile: manual of directions. Institute of Rehabilitation Medicine, New York University Medical Center, New York, 1969.
59. Sarno, J. E., Sarno, M. T. & Levita, E.: The Functional Life Scale. Arch Phys Med Rehab 54: 214, 1973.
60. Schuell, H.: The Minnesota Test for Differential Diagnosis of Aphasia. University of Minnesota Press, Minneapolis, 1965.
61. Schuell, H., Jenkins, J. & Jimenez-Pabon, E.: Aphasia in Adults. Harper & Row, New York, 1964.
62. Shankweiler, D. & Harris, K.: An experimental approach to the problems of articulation in aphasia. Cortex 2: 277, 1966.
63. Shewan, C. & Canter, G.: Effects of vocabulary, syntax, and sentence length on auditory comprehension in aphasic patients. Cortex 7: 209, 1971.
64. Spreen, O.: Language disturbances in cerebrovascular disease. In: A. L. Benton (ed.), Behavioral Changes in Cerebrovascular Disease, pp. 40–45. Harper & Row, New York, 1970.
65. Spreen, O. & Benton, A. L.: Neurosensory Center Comprehensive Examination for Aphasia: manual of directions. Neuropsychology Laboratory, University of Victoria, Victoria, B.C., 1969.
66. Strubb, R. & Gardner, H.: Repetition deficit viewed as linguistic deficit—specifically in the processing, synthesis and ordering of phonemes. Brain Lang 1: 241, 1974.
67. Taylor, M. L.: A measurement of functional communication in aphasia. Arch Phys Med Rehab 46: 101, 1965.
68. Wagenaar, E., Snow, C. & Prins, R.: Spontaneous speech of aphasic patients: a psycholinguistic analysis. Brain Lang 2: 281, 1975.
69. Weisenberg, T. & McBride, K.: Aphasia: A Clinical and Psychological Study. Hafner, New York, 1964. (First edition: Commonwealth Fund, 1935.)
70. Wepman, J. & Jones, L.: Studies in Aphasia: An Approach to Testing—Manual of Administration and Scoring for the Language Modalities Test for Aphasia. Educational Industry Service, Chicago, 1961.
71. Wepman, J. & Jones, L.: Studies in aphasia: classification of aphasic speech by noun–pronoun ratio. Br J Dis Communic 1: 46, 1966.
72. Yamadori, A. & Albert, M.: Word category aphasia. Cortex 9: 112, 1973.
73. Yarnell, P., Monroe, P. & Sobel, L.: Aphasia outcome in stroke: a clinical neuro-radiological correlation. Stroke 7: 514, 1976.

Aphasia rehabilitation

MARTHA TAYLOR SARNO

In the section which reviewed recovery and rehabilitation in aphasia certain social and medical currents were described which led directly to the demand for aphasia remediation. This demand has grown steadily over the years and with it there has been a proliferation of treatment methods. As with classification and testing, therapeutic approaches have been based upon theoretical concepts of the nature of language and pathology of aphasia. It is, therefore, not possible to classify therapeutic methods in any logical way. What follows will be a somewhat random presentation of some of the main trends of aphasia therapy.

Wepman and Schuell

Wepman (63, 64) presented one of the first elaborations of a therapeutic approach the goal of which was to "stimulate" language in the aphasic patient. He suggested that the manner of stimuli presentation was of paramount importance and that it was not the role of the therapist to teach vocabulary or syntax. One of the techniques he suggested was the presentation of film strips selected for individual patients according to their levels of interest and competence (67). A stimulation approach was also developed by Schuell and her associates (44) who stated, "in our opinion the clinician's role is not that of a teacher. He has nothing to do with teaching the adult aphasic to talk or to read or to write. He does not teach the patient sounds or rules for combining words. Rather he tries to communicate with the patient and stimulate disrupted processes to function maximally." A key principle is that "It would seem that sensory stimulation is the only method we have for making complex events happen in the brain. That stimulus must be adequate and it must get into the brain. It involves repetitive sensory stimulation, each stimulus eliciting a response" (8).

Most aphasia therapists today provide therapy based on the work of Wepman or Schuell. To elaborate further, though both of these leaders emphasized the importance of stimulation in therapy, Schuell was more specific as to the procedures which should be employed.

Her approach, one of the most detailed in the field of aphasia therapy, is based on the premise that auditory processing impairments underlie aphasia. She stressed adequate stimulation, carefully controlled for length, rate and loudness. She saw individual therapy as more effective than group therapy because of the individual differences among patients and their deficits. Within her framework, one language modality is used to stimulate another in a program carefully graded for complexity. She stressed the importance of repetition and overt responses from patients with a minimum of correcting or explaining on the part of the therapist. Schuell saw the treatment atmosphere as very important in its ability to increase the patient's self-esteem. The importance of establishing rapport was also a major focus of Schuell. However, since none of these variables has been submitted to rigorous study, the extent of their importance is not known. Her approach to aphasia therapy is elaborated in her book (44).

Wepman held to the view that there were no specific formulae to be followed in administering treatment for aphasia, that the efforts should be stimulating, indirect, not focused on specific behaviors. He stated, "Therapy under the suggested regimen should center on the patient's thought processes by extending content and substance. Topics known to be of interest to the patient from his pre-traumatic life history should be elaborated largely through an increased focus on visualization. Stimulation remains the core of therapy with ideas presented both verbally and nonverbally. No attempt to produce specific words or controlled syntax are made—rather whatever is produced is accepted as the patient's best possible response at the moment" (65).

In later writings Wepman proposed the thesis that language is inseparably related to thought but not identical with it ... that it is the product of thought and the maidservant of man's highest mental processing. He saw the process of stimulation in speech therapy as an "embellishment of thought"—removing the implied criticism of corrective therapy—never asking for or trying in any way to elicit verbal expression (66).

Wepman continued to reject the notion of aphasia as a specific speech or language disorder and interpreted the disturbance as a "disorder affecting the patient's total reaction pattern due to a disturbance of the integrating capacity of the cortex". His "indirect" stimulation approach was the natural result of his views on the nature of the disorder. He saw direct psycholinguistic attacks on the aphasic manifestation as most likely to become rigid language approaches, and placed a premium on innovation, ingenuity, and individual creativity in therapy with aphasic patients.

In the case of patients with phonetic impairment, Wepman (66) and many others (33, 38, 39, 44) have recommended direct methods of articulation therapy along traditional lines in which the basis is primarily imitation practice with visual and kinesthetic cues.

The possibility that linguistic principles might apply to re-education in aphasia has been raised by a number of authors (24, 34, 35, 42, 52, 55) presented a theoretical orientation toward language reacquisition for aphasic adults on the basis of what is known about neurological, linguistic, and psycholinguistic aspects of natural language. More recently Ludlow (29) observed that there was a common order of recovery of syntactic structures in the aphasics she studied, regardless of type of aphasia or whether or not they were treated. She suggested that the same syntactic sequence might provide a logical basis for a treatment regimen.

Hundreds of specific techniques have been mentioned in the aphasia literature including practice in reading aloud (46); structured conversational practice (7); role-playing, pantomine and impersonation (43); and social group programs (2, 3). Some have advocated concentrating on vocabulary building around common themes (e.g., house furnishings) (1, 53).

Goldstein (13) and Lenneberg (29) felt that the therapist might help the patient to compensate for impaired function. They claimed, in fact, that the patient could develop these himself as a result of the tendency of most organisms to come into the best possible condition despite a remaining defect.

Wiegel-Crump (68) studied two treatment methods (programmed and non-structured) with the goal of increasing syntax retrieval. After four weeks of highly structured therapy, improvement in syntax generation did not generalize from specific items drilled on in therapy to additional non-drilled items. The level of improvement on non-drilled items did not significantly differ from the level of improvement on drilled items.

Hatfield and Zangwill (15) employed a picture story method in which the capacity of aphasic patients to communicate a sequence of events by drawing was explored. The idea is that ideational processes in aphasia may be substantially intact in spite of severe defects in speaking and writing.

Luria (30) used a "card index plan" to train a post-traumatic, mildly impaired aphasic who had difficulty in producing fluent narrative speech. The patient was trained to write down, on separate cards, fragments of the theme he was to relate, and to speak from them. Luria's idea was that a defective internal system can be replaced by an external aid and in this instance writing was used to facilitate speech.

Beyn & Shokhor-Troskaya (5) reported on the effect of a specific plan of therapy with 25 post stroke patients. They attempted to "prevent the appearance of some of the speech defects of aphasic patients which, up to now, seemed to be inevitable", specifically "telegraphic style" of responses. They avoided teaching nominative words, teaching at first only simple words which could function as a whole sentence—words like "no, there, here, give, tomorrow, and thanks". Only when words appeared spontaneously in a patient's speech were nouns introduced into therapy. These were never introduced in the nominative case but only in one of the other five Russian cases involving some inflection. "The results of the rehabilitation of active speech varied; but the most important fact is that telegraphic style, which is inevitable with other methods of rehabilitation, did not emerge in any of our patients".

Behavior modification

The application of the principles of behavior modification to aphasia therapy is a good example of method following theoretical concept. It was perhaps inevitable that an attempt would be made to apply the work of B. F. Skinner to the problem of aphasia therapy. Let us first consider operant conditioning. The use of operant conditioning rests on the asumption that the desired behavior, or a behavior similar to it, exists in the patient's behavioral inventory and can be manipulated so that it will occur in a specifiable manner in response to a specific stimulus. The assumption is supported by several studies, although Lenneberg (28) thought that aphasia was not a learning impairment, and that conditioning procedures should not be effective in restoring language to a patient with a well-established aphasia.

Tikofsky and Reynolds (56) found that conditioning occurred in aphasic subjects, but more slowly than in normal subjects. Goodkin (14) reported that verbal perseveration and inappropriateness were altered in two aphasic subjects. Jacobs and Taylor (23) reported that an aphasic who had been in treatment for seven years was able to increase and maintain her verb repertoire as a result of an experiment using poker chips as reinforcement, and Lane and Moore (27) successfully conditioned aphasics who could not discriminate between the phonemes [t] and [d].

Smith (48) studied operant conditioning of syntax in aphasia in a 32 year old patient who was 6 months post and a 65 year old 11 months post stroke. Using an informal, operant conditioning technique which did not require the patient to speak, and a two-stage training procedure, the subject was taught to use prepositions and word-order to convey the nature and direction of a spatial relationship. The two patients learned to choose prepositions that correctly identified spatial relationships among objects. They learned sequencing strategy which enabled them to arrange three word cards to describe an object display. The patients learned what they could not do spontaneously. The results of this work may suggest the successful use of conditioning techniques to enable non-language mechanisms to solve, or help solve, language problems.

Behavioral strategies in aphasia therapy show concern for careful delineation and measurement of the desired end-point behaviors.

Holland (17) discusses the nature of reinforcers one uses along the way, and most important, the need for careful attention to gradually changing either the topography of the behavior in question or to systematically altering the stimulus conditions in which the desired behavior is supposed to occur—the process of successive approximation in clinical application.

The programmed instruction approach views language rehabilitation as an educative process and applies, in a rigorous way, operant conditioning methods drawn from learning theory and principles drawn from psycholinguistic analysis to guide the content and order of presentation of the linguistic elements taught (17, 18, 52). It is based on the belief that there are several distinguishable stages of learning, including recognition, imitation, repetition of the model based on memory of the echoed performance, and finally, spontaneous selection of a response from a repertoire of learned responses (7).

Many types of materials requiring aphasics to perform a variety of tasks on automated devices has suggested that even severely impaired aphasics can learn to match visual configurations, to perform visual oddity tasks, and to write their names. Rosenberg (37) used automated training procedures in an experiment designed to assess and train aphasics to make perceptual discriminations basic to reading. These programs were effective in teaching such discriminations as well as in increasing the rate of response and retention of the material. Edwards (9) investigated differential responses to tasks involving the matching of visual stimuli by more than 100 severely impaired aphasics and found that all but 4 of the patients successfully completed the program. In still another study, Filby and Edwards (10) taught form discrimination to 12 severely impaired aphasics and 10 normal subjects. In the optimal learning conditions of the experiment, the aphasic group did not differ significantly from the controls; they also did not exhibit "catastrophic" reactions or other forms of disruptive responses.

Holland and Levy (19) have expressed the behavioristic view that aphasics learn by having consequences applied to their behavior and that the clinician's primary concern should be to screen subject matter and control reinforcement. Making this possible is the outgrowth of operant conditioning which is called programmed instruction. Based on the premise that aphasic patients need smaller steps, more than an average number of repetitions, and a more systematically structured teaching procedure (51, 53, 54) the technology of programmed instruction lends itself to experimentation with these patients.

Holland and Sonderman (20) attempted to teach 24 aphasic patients tasks from the *Token Test* (TT) in a programmed approach. Patients had a mean age of 54.5 years and a mean time since onset of 5.6 years. All patients except two head trauma patients had aphasia secondary to CVA. Patients were rated on a severity scale as follows: 4 mild, 6 mild-moderate, 5 moderate, 3 moderate-severe, and 6 severe. They were divided into low and high groups according to TT scores. As a result of the training, the mild and mild-moderate patients demonstrated significant improvement while the moderate and severe patients did not. In addition, the high group was more receptive to the program than the low group. Training was most effective for those who initially did well, however, no patient was error free. In general, the patients did not easily transfer language skills acquired in the program to similar untrained tasks.

In a kind of re-vamping of a traditional approach Weigl (60, 61) developed an approach to therapy called "deblocking" which is based on the factor of context. It is essentially a systematic use of a patients intact modalities. For example, if a patient is having trouble with auditory recognition, he may be helped in his recognition of a given word by having pre-stimulation with the same stimulus through the visual channel. Deblocking seems to be naturally in tune with clinical approaches which build new responses upon a patient's most intact language skill. The clearest clinical description of deblocking therapy is in a longitudinal report of Ulatowska and Richardson (57).

Ulatowska and Richardson (57) used a deblocking technique to reintegrate the mechanisms for correlating sound and meaning with adult aphasic patients with severe impairment of auditory comprehension. The visual mode of presentation of linguistic material was used both to provide a stable representation of speech units and to allow reinforcement of auditory representations. The patient was given tasks of repetition, reading aloud, and sequencing, using progressively more complex material. The behavior of the patient gives support to the viability of the theoretical constructs of lingustics: this can be seen in the differential processing of function words vs. content words, and in the orderly progression of improvement through stages explicable as the recovery of well-defined and hierarchically dependent subcomponents of linguistic organization.

Each word of a phrase was printed on a card. The patient was instructed to arrange the cards in proper sequence. This was followed by having the patient:

1. Match phrase to an appropriate picture (reading comprehension).
2. Point to appropriate phrase on command (facilitating auditory recognition of longer words with visual presentations).
3. Point to each component word on command (auditory understanding of units in a phrase).
4. Point to picture on command (auditory recognition without written word).
5. Listen to phrase as read by clinician (auditory stimulation).
6. Answer simple questions pertaining to the phrase, by pointing to the correct card (understanding of both the phrase and its components).

Overall improvement was reported in:

1. Comprehension of language (if spoken slowly in relatively concrete sentences with frequent repetitions).
2. Auditory retention of three words.
3. Recognition of language errors.
4. Comprehension of reading material (restricted to a one sentence span of four to six words).
5. Repetition of single words.
6. Decrease of jargon.
7. Retrieval of words.
8. Spontaneous writing of name and numbers.
9. Copying sentences.
10. Improved gestures.

There was no improvement noted in:

1. Comprehension of complex reading material (lengthy involved sentences or paragraphs).
2. Spontaneous writing of single words.

Three recent methods bear special mention. The first of these is identified by the acronym VIC, which stands for Visual Communication Therapy (12).

The method, intended for the global aphasic, was modeled after work done by Premack (36) who reported an experiment in which a chimpanzee was taught a simple communication system. VIC employs an index card system of arbitrary symbols representing syntactic and lexical components. Patients learn to recognize the symbols and manipulate them so as to (1) respond to a command, (2) answer a question relative to the circumstance, (3) describe actions, and (4) express needs, wishes or other emotions. It attempts to circumvent the use of natural oral language which is so severely impaired in the global aphasic patient.

The program includes two levels of communicative functions. At Level 1 patients carry out commands, answer questions, and describe actions; at Level 2, they employ the system spontaneously to express desires and feelings.

Of 8 patients given sufficient opportunity to master VIC, 5 completed Level 1, and 2 of these also satisfied the criteria for Level 2. Among these 5 patients, performance in VIC far surpassed performance on matching tasks in English, error rates were quite low and the pattern of errors was remarkably similar. An inverse correlation was obtained between ability in English and in the use of VIC.

The evidence suggests that some severely aphasic patients can master the basics of an alternative symbol system. Moreover several indices suggest that the communicative consequences of the system are appreciated, and that at least some of the cognitive operations entailed in natural language persist despite severe aphasia.

In personal communication with these experimenters, they have expressed the idea that the method may have more relevance as a means of exploring residual mental function in global aphasics than as a system of therapy.

Sparks, Helm and Albert (50) described a therapeutic regimen called Melodic Intonation Therapy (MIT) based upon the observation that language which is unavailable in spontaneous speech can sometimes be produced in association with a sung melody. The system presumes an intact right hemisphere, thought to be the locus of melodic production. It proceeds on the assumption that functional language can be developed if it is "taught" in association with rhythm and melody. In a series of carefully graded steps the therapist slowly introduces melody, rhythm and verbal content, gradually including the patient in the process and eventually leaving the patient as the sole "performer".

In the experience of the authors, success is more likely in patients who fulfill the following criteria:

1. Good auditory comprehension.
2. Facility for self-correction.
3. Markedly limited verbal output.
4. Reasonably good attention span.
5. Good emotional stability (16, 32).

Sparks and his colleagues have suggested that the system "deblocks" spoken language for patients with good auditory comprehension. On the whole, MIT has resulted in clearcut generalized language gains for aphasics meeting the above description who have previously demonstrated little or no change with more traditional therapy.

Programming principles were applied to MIT because they insured that the procedure would move slowly, could be explicitly communicated to others and requires systematic data collection which could be used to determine the success of the approach.

The third of these recently introduced therapeutic techniques is somewhat parallel to MIT. Skelley et al. (47, 48) employed Amerind (American Indian Sign Language) in an attempt to facilitate articulatory efficiency in patients with severe speech dyspraxia (cortical dysarthria.). As melody is used to facilitate verbal production in global aphasics, this method explores the value of systematized gestural language to improve oral production. For the purposes of this method the authors modified Amerind and a programmed system was developed in which signs are taught first, then associated with the corresponding vocal and oral processes. The authors reported modest success.

The foregoing review of therapeutic techniques was not intended to be exhaustive. For those interested in a more complete review the author's chapter in the book *Communication Disorders* (41) is recommended.

Toward a comprehensive view of Aphasia rehabilitation

In my view, aphasia rehabilitation is a process of patient management in the broadest sense. The impact of aphasia, mild or severe, is far reaching and affects all aspects of life in important ways. To be effective aphasia rehabilitation must combine social, psychological, linguistic and all other "therapies" into a cohesive regimen. It is difficult to imagine that any speech therapy technique could represent the total answer to a condition as catastrophically all-encompassing as aphasia.

The holistic approach to therapeutic intervention which is traditionally practiced in the rehabilitation medicine setting seems essential to the goal of maximizing a patient's residual verbal abilities. Effective aphasia rehabilitation is a total management process in which speech therapy, in the sense of the application of remediation techniques, is essential and important but not exclusively responsible for optimal outcome.

First and foremost, one must acknowledge and have full understanding of the uniqueness of the individual aphasic patient. This is not simply to pay lip service to the humanistic idea that we are all created differently but to recognize in the fullest sense that no two aphasic persons are exactly alike in pathology, personality, linguistic deficits, reactions to catastrophic illness, spiritual values, etc. Further, that the influence of these factors assumes different characteristics and strength at different states of recovery and that they are all inextricably related to recovery outcome.

A stroke usually marks a dramatic turning point in a patient's life. It arrives "unheralded and unannounced" (58). In one sense, the patient's premorbid personality is all important. It forms the nexus out of which all subsequent adaptive responses arrive. Most commonly what occurs is an accentuation of underlying trends in the premorbid personality coming into focus (58).

Certain reactions are repeatedly cited as characteristic of the early stages of aphasia. Many patients experience a "vague", "grey", dreamlike state coupled with a lack of interest in surroundings and a lack of concern or awareness of what has happened. The duration of this state is widely variable. Once the patient begins to be aware and take interest in his environment other reactions which have a marked influence on recovery become apparent. These include the loss of self-esteem, loneliness, isolation, anger, anxiety, frustration, and fear. Although some bear the ravages of stroke with equanimity others are thrown into a deep depression. Ullman observed that the variability of reactions is rarely determined by the type or location of lesion but is an expression of the whole life experience of the person who has had a stroke (58). The following are some relevant direct quotations from his writing:

... the need to focus not on an abstract appraisal of psychopathological patterns but on understanding the current life situation and the consequent meaning of the stroke to the patient at this particular moment in his life. Repeatedly one gets the feeling in talking with these patients that had the stroke occurred a year or two earlier or a year or two later, their reactions would have been quite different. At times it climaxes a process of resignation and surrender set in motion years before; at other times it initiates such a process. In some patients it touches off a last-ditch stand dedicated to the pursuit of unattained life goals and ambitions. Occasionally it opens up new vistas for the elaboration of secondary gain from illness. Unrealistic strivings for independence and unrealistic dependency are perhaps the two main channels into which irrational modes of adaptation flow.

Although reactive in nature, the depressions experienced by stroke patients differ in several respects from the usual type of depression. The varied and overwhelming life problems confronting these patients make it difficult to distinguish realistically rooted feelings of resignation, futility and despair from more neurotically patterned reactions. On several occasions the depression seemed to be associated with the premonition of imminent demise which, at times, proved a more accurate prognostic indicator than the objective medical estimate of the facts. Is it neurotic to wish to give up the struggle when the odds are genuinely against the person involved? This is the question posed by the type of depression often experienced by stroke patients. In one way or another the depression calls attention to the real suffering associated with physical incapacity and deterioration, loneliness, abandonment and neglect (both familial and social). Not infrequently, the depressive affect is masked by stoical attitudes or simply by the absorption of the individual in habitual and automatic patterns of behavior.

In personal accounts of aphasia patients often describe the correlation between increased awareness of impairment and depressions. Guy Wint (69) a British journalist who wrote a book about his stroke said, "My outlook darkened and was markedly more gloomy after two years than it had been in the early part of the illness. I found a general gloom congenial. I preferred night to daylight, autumn to spring, sad stories to comedy, the end of things to their cheerful beginning." He also writes, "I shall never forget the feeling of despair and annoyance that arose in me when my doctor said: 'You are perfectly allright now'."

Several authors have recognized the importance of defense mechanisms in the individual's reaction to catastrophic illness (4, 11, 21, 25, 26, 59, 62). These reactions are essentially natural attempts to ward off depression and anxiety and postpone the acknowledgement of chronic illness. Baretz and Stephenson (4) felt that denial allows the patient to "borrow time" to deal with the depression that would overwhelm him if he accepted the disability and its implications.

Denial may manifest itself by overoptimism and unusual confidence, often reflected in "(1) understanding the physical disability and its permanence, hence, denying the need for treatment, or (2) overestimating the ability to recover, resulting in demanding behavior and anger at the staff for not doing enough to cure the disability."

Some problems that arise when one uses the term denial were raised by Ullman and Gruen (59) in connection with patients who have sustained brain damage. In traditional psychiatric usage the term refers to a specific psycho-dynamic mechanism designed to influence the demands of the interpersonal situation in which an individual protects himself by pushing the pain of a particular situation out of awareness. In the case of the brain damaged patient Ullman and Gruen felt that the patient does not use denial as a psychodynamic mechanism but as a convenient way of explaining certain reactions. He encounters difficulty in relating to the deficit because of his incapacity to be aware of the defect and not an awareness that is suppressed in the service of avoiding anxiety. What emerges as apparent denial is the effort to cover up the areas of unawareness as these are encroached upon by the environment. The anxiety level becomes a function of the relative success the patient has in covering up or avoiding involvement in the deficit. Horenstein (22) interprets denial as an extension of the patient's prior personality. That is, those who employ denial as a defense in the post stroke state are often those who solved problems by denial before the stroke. Ullman (58) commented that these defenses exist in proportion to what is at stake: that those with more to lose, especially the younger and more active are more likely to resort to denial than the older patient who has already made an adjustment to reduced activity imposed by advancing years.

In a study of aphasic patients participating in a group psychotherapy program Friedman (11) investigated the nature of psychological regression in aphasia. He felt that beyond the actual communication difficulties posed by aphasia, in the patients he studied there was a sense that each patient remained psychologically an individual island. They did not maintain a consistent level of group participation and expressed intense feelings that they were very different from other people. Both withdrawal and projection were apparent as each patient acted in isolation and yet complained of this characteristic in others. His study suggested that aphasia can result in regressive behavior with impaired reality testing. Patients made a defensive use of dependence as manifested in a recurring demand that they be given more help by the therapist and preferably in smaller groups where individualized attention would be provided (11).

Clearly, the magnitude and complexity of the psychosocial aspects of aphasia are considerable. Some have worked directly with these facets of the patient's behavior in a modified version of psychotherapy (2, 6). The impact on all interpersonal relationships in and out of the family needs little elaboration. It is understandable that some efforts have been directed solely at counseling and educating families of aphasic patients since the family in the final analysis is left with the ultimate responsibility for the patient's welfare (31, 39, 51).

The process of aphasia rehabilitation is one of participating with the individual patient in working through the evolution of emotional and adaptive phases which are in many ways inseparable from linguistic recovery. One of the most effective management tools is the selective and discriminating use of speech therapy to stimulate and support the patient through the various stages of recovery.

Speech therapy serves different purposes at different points along the way. Sometimes it helps the patient to "borrow time" as Baretz and Stephenson (4) so aptly stated. At other times it helps him assess his linguistic strengths and weaknesses and test these against reality expectations. The observation that a depression often lifts after speech therapy has been initiated may be more a response to the supportive and nurturing nature of the therapeutic relationship rather than any objective improvement in speech (58).

Viewed this way aphasia rehabilitation can be understood as a dynamic process consisting of a series of stages through which the majority of patients evolve. Some patients, of course, never move from the first stage and remain seriously depressed.

In her classic characterization of the stages of death and dying Elizabeth Kuebler-Ross (25) provides a good model for describing the recovery phases in aphasia. She specifies five stages: Denial and Isolation; Anger; Bargaining; Depression; and Acceptance.

In recovery from aphasia I should like to identify three stages: Depression/denial, Anger, and Adaptation. Enlightened aphasia management is responsive to the patients recovery states and linguistic evolution.

In the first stage the patient usually withdraws from friends and social situations, he is lethargic, often complains about chronic fatigue and manifests all of the universal signs of hopelessness. He may make unrealistic plans based on complete recovery, set deadline dates for recovery, or otherwise stall for time while the depression resolves. Health professionals are generally poorly equipped to deal with these behaviors. They are usually unaccepting of these symptoms as the natural consequences of chronic disease and tend to express anger at the patient's "unrealistic attitude".

Their anger becomes aggravated by the frustration and failure inherent in trying to bring the patient closer to a realistic attitude. Therapists are not generally kindly disposed to patients who are preoccupied and self-involved, seclusive, or express hopeless attitudes.

The speech therapy process serves an important purpose during this stage. By directly addressing the patient's linguistic deficits and channeling attention and energies toward constructive ends, there can sometimes be a noticeable reduction in depressive reactions. Speech therapy, in this instance, may act as an equivalent for work which has long been recognized as an antidote for depression. The title of a chapter written in a personal account of a stroke patient (70): "My Lifeline to Sanity, The Marvels of Speech Therapy" is a powerful testament to the psychological impact of speech therapy.

Certain principles were suggested by Baretz and Stephenson (4) as guidelines in the management of the patient who is unrealistic which seem worthy of citing here since they can be used as a basis for speech therapy.

1. Provide appropriate information to the patient. Evasiveness can arouse deeper fears or delay acceptance. Information for the family is equally important lest they undermine the patient's acceptance of reality by expressing their own unrealistic goals.
2. Stress functioning rather than recovery.
3. Allow some hope, for motivation. Whereas the staff tends to regard the patient's unrealistic attitudes as a threat to potential adjustment, the patient often needs to retain some hope to avoid yielding to depression.
4. Permit the patient to test his fantasied capacity.
5. Allow the patient some sense of control.

Staff members tend to reject the unrealistic demands of patients as manipulative. Working with the patient as a partner, allowing him to channel his initative into planning his program constructively helps restore feelings of self worth.

In his book *Autobiographical Considerations on Aphasia Rehabilitation* Dr Renato Segre recommends that there is some value to allowing the patient to delay speaking and to economize on the length and complexity of utterances. He says "It is important not to interrupt these resting periods because they represent a defense and compensation measure ... some aphasics enjoy their verbal silence. It is a kind of spiritual rest, of quiet criticism on other people's opinions; a kind of personal formula to reach a better optimism" (45).

In the second stage, the anger which the patient originally directed toward himself is now outwardly directed. Some patients act out by physical means or by confrontations with family or staff members. During this stage the patient is particularly difficult to manage. By understanding this phase as a natural and necessary part of the recovery course those around the patient can continue to provide a supportive environment.

The third and last stage is a period of adaptation which continues for the remainder of the patient's life. It is in this period that the patient mobilizes and brings to bear all of his strengths and begins to compensate for losses. In the post stroke patient the pattern of linguistic impairment is stabilized by one year after onset and although improvement continues indefinitely beyond this period, full recovery in all communication skills is rare if not achieved by this time.

The speech pathologist who is attuned to the psychological evolution of recovery from aphasia applies an armamentarium of therapeutic approaches which takes the recovery phases into account and tries to maximize the characteristics and needs according to the particular recovery stage.

Group speech therapy, stroke clubs, and other social groups, for example, are techniques which are frequently employed in the management of patients with chronic aphasia. They serve their best function after the acute and spontaneous recovery periods when the patient is generally more aware of his deficits, and less preoccupied with symptoms. By this time the patient is beginning to be interested in and capable of interacting with others. He can gain support from other patients by sharing feelings with those who have gone through the same experience. Knowledge that one is not alone usually helps to reduce depression and loneliness.

The late Hildred Schuell was always especially concerned with the humanitarian aspects of aphasia rehabilitation. I would like to conclude my comments with a quotation from her book (44) as follows:

There has always been a good deal of discussion about the art and the science of professions that include clinical practice as well as laboratory research. If by art one means appreciation of the fact that one is dealing with human life, and by science one means precise information, both are necessary and must go hand in hand. In a sense they have always done so. This is to say that asking questions and making observations is not the exclusive domain of either art or science, or the clinic or the laboratory. The dichotomy seems to reflect the either-orishness that Aristotelian language habits have tended to impose on our thinking. What the clinican cannot get along without, and what great artists and scientists alike have always had, is a kind of reverence for human life. The great literature of all times and places has had something to say about the human condition as searching and as probing as the questions scientists have asked about the nature of the universe and the nature of man. Scientists have learned that one cannot leave the observer out of the equation, and clinicians know one cannot leave the laboratory out of the clinic.

References

1. Agranowitz, A. & McKeown, M.: Aphasia Handbook for Adults and Children. Edwards Brothers, Ann Arbor, 1959.
2. Aronson, M., Shatin, L. & Cook, J.: Socio-psychotherapeutic approach to the treatment of aphasic patients. J Speech Hear Dis 21: 352, 1956.

3. Backus, O. L.: The use of a group structure in speech therapy. J Speech Hear Dis 17: 116, 1952.
4. Baretz, R. & Stephenson, G.: Unrealistic patient. N Y State J Med 54, 1976.
5. Beyn, E. & Shokhor-Trotskaya, M.: The preventive method of speech rehabilitation in aphasia. Cortex 2: 96, 1966.
6. Blackman, N.: Group psychotherapy with aphasics. J Neuro Ment Dis 111: 154, 1950.
7. Boone, D.: A plan for rehabilitation of aphasic patients. Arch Phys Med Rehab 48: 410, 1967.
8. Darley, F. L.: The efficacy of language rehabilitation in aphasia. J Speech Hear Dis 37: 3, 1972.
9. Edwards, A.: Automated training for a "matching-to-sample" task in aphasia. J Speech Hear Res 8: 39, 1965.
10. Filby, Y. & Edwards, A.: An application of automated-teaching methods to test and teach form discrimination to aphasics. J Prog Instruc 2: 25, 1963.
11. Friedman, M.: On the nature of regression. Arch Gen Psychiat 5: 60, 1961.
12. Gardner, H., Zurif, E., Berry, T. & Baker, E.: Visual communication in aphasia. Neuropsychologia 14: 275, 1976.
13. Goldstein, K.: Language and Language Disturbances. Grune & Stratton, New York, 1948.
14. Goodkin, R.: Use of concurrent response categories in evaluating talking behavior in aphasic patients. Percept Motor Skills 26: 1035, 1968.
15. Hatfield, F. & Zangwill, O.: Ideation in aphasia: the picture story method. Neuropsychologia 12: 389, 1974.
16. Helm, N.: Assessing candidacy for melodic intonation therapy. Paper presented at American Speech and Hearing Association Convention, Texas, 1976.
17. Holland, A.: Some current trends in aphasia rehabilitation. ASHA 11: 3, 1969.
18. Holland, A.: Case studies in aphasia rehabilitation using programmed instruction. J Speech Hear Res 35: 377, 1970.
19. Holland, A. & Levy, C.: Syntactic gerneralization in aphasics as a function of relearning an active sentence. Acta Symbol 2: 34, 1971.
20. Holland, A. & Sonderman, J.: Effects of a program based on the Token Test for teaching comprehension skills to aphasics. J Speech Hear Res 17: 589, 1974.
21. Hook, O.: Neuropsychological aspects of motivation. Scand J Rehab Med 8: 97, 1976.
22. Horenstein, S.: Presentation 17. In: A. L. Benton (ed.), Behavioral Changes in Cerebrovascular Disease. Harper & Row, New York, 1970.
23. Jacobs, C. & Taylor, M. L.: The application of operant conditioning techniques to aphasia therapy. Paper presented at American Speech and Hearing Association Convention, Washington, D.C., 1966.
24. Jakobson, R.: Aphasia as a linguistic problem. In: H. Werner (ed.), On Expressive Language, pp. 69–81. Clark University Press, Worcester, Mass., 1955.
25. Keubler-Ross, E.: On Death and Dying. MacMillan, New York, 1969.
26. Krupp, N.: Psychiatric implications of chronic and crippling illness. Psychosomatics 9: 109, 1968.
27. Lane, H. & Moore, D.: Reconditioning a consonant discrimination in an aphasic: an experimental case history. J Speech Hear Dis 27: 232, 1962.
28. Lenneberg, E.: Biological Foundations of Language. Wiley & Sons, New York, 1967.
29. Ludlow, C.: Recovery from aphasia: a foundation for treatment. In: M. Sullivan & M. Krommers (eds.), Rationale for Adult Aphasia Therapy, pp. 97–134. University of Nebraska Medical Center, Omaha, 1977.

30. Luria, A. R.: Human Brain and Psychological Processes. Harper & Row, New York, 1966.
31. Malone, R.: Expressed attitudes of families of aphasics. J Speech Hear Dis 34: 146, 1969.
32. Marshall, N. & Holtzapple, P.: Melodic intonation therapy: variations on a theme. In: R. Brookshire (ed.), Clinical Aphasiology—Conference Proceedings. BRK Pub., Minneapolis, 1976.
33. Millikan, C. & Darley, F. L.: Brain Mechanisms Underlying Speech and Language. Grune & Stratton, New York, 1967.
34. Morley, H.: Applying linguistics to speech and language therapy for aphasics. Lang Learn 10: 135, 1960.
35. Pincas, A.: Linguistics and aphasia. J Australian Coll Speech Ther 15: 20, 1965.
36. Premack, D.: Language in chimpanzee? Science 172: 808, 1971.
37. Rosenberg, B.: The performance of aphasics on automated visuo-perceptual discrimination, training and transfer tasks. J Speech Hear Res 8: 165, 1965.
38. Sarno, J. E. & Sarno, M. T.: The diagnosis of speech disorders in brain damaged adults. Med Clin N America 53: 561, 1969.
39. Sarno, J. E. & Sarno, M. T.: Stroke: The Condition and the Patient. McGraw-Hill, New York, 1969, 2nd edition, 1979.
40. Sarno, M. T.: The role of the family in aphasia. In: T. Hanley (ed.), The Family as Supportive Personnel in Speech and Hearing Remediation: Proceedings of the Post-Graduate Course, pp. 61–66. University of California, California, 1971.
41. Sarno, M. T.: Aphasia rehabilitation. In: S. Dickson (ed.), Communication Disorders: Remedial Principles and Practices, pp. 399–440. Scott, Foresman, Glenview, Ill., 1974.
42. Scargill, M.: Modern linguistics and recovery from aphasia. J Speech Hear Dis 19: 507, 1964.
43. Schlanger, P. & Schlanger, B.: Adapting role-playing activities with aphasic patients. J Speech Hear Dis 35: 229, 1970.
44. Schuell, H., Jenkins, J. & Jimenez-Pabon, E.: Aphasia in Adults. Harper & Row, New York, 1964.
45. Segre, R.: Autobiographical considerations on aphasic rehabilitation. Folia Phoniat 28: 129, 1976.
46. Sheehan, V.: Techniques in the management of aphasics. J Speech Hear Dis 13: 241, 1948.
47. Skelly, M., Schinsky, L., Smith, R., Donaldson, R. & Griffin, J.: American Indian sign: a gestural communication system for the speechless. Arch Phys Med Rehab 56: 156, 1975.
48. Skelly, M., Schinsky, L., Smith, R. & Fust, R.: American Indian sign (AMERIND) as a facilitator of verbalization for the oral verbal apraxic. J Speech Hear Dis 39: 445, 1974.
49. Smith, M.: Operant conditioning of syntax in aphasia. Neuropsychologia 12: 403, 1974.
50. Sparks, R., Helm, N. & Albert, M.: Aphasia rehabilitation resulting from melodic intonation therapy. Cortex 10: 303, 1974.
51. Taylor, M. L.: Language therapy. In Burr, H. (ed.), The Aphasic Adult: Evaluation and Rehabilitation. Proceedings of a Short Course in Aphasia, pp. 139–160. University of Virginia, Wayside, Charlottesville, 1964.
52. Taylor, M. L.: Linguistic considerations of the verbal behavior of brain damaged adults. Ling Rep 6: 1, 1964.
53. Taylor, M. L. & Marks, M.: Aphasia Rehabilitation Manual and Therapy Kit. McGraw-Hill, New York, 1959.

54. Taylor, M. L. & Sands, E.: Application of programmed instruction techniques to the language rehabilitation of severely impaired aphasic patients. Nat Soc Prog Instruc J 5: 10, 1966.
55. Taylor, O. & Anderson, C.: Neuropsycholinguistics and language training. Paper presented at Congress on Language Retraining for Aphasics. Ohio State University, 1968.
56. Tikofsky, R. & Reynolds, G.: Further studies of non-verbal learning and aphasia. J Speech Hear Res 6: 133, 1963.
57. Ulatowska, H. & Richardson, S.: A longitudinal study of an adult with aphasia: considerations for research and therapy. Brain Lang 1: 151, 1974.
58. Ullman, M.: Behavioral Changes in Patients Following Strokes. Charles C. Thomas, Springfield, Ill., 1962.
59. Ullman, M. & Greun, A.: Behavioral changes in patients with strokes. Am J Psychiat 117: 1004, 1961.
60. Weigl, E.: The phenomenon of temporary deblocking in aphasia. Zeitschrift für Phonetik, Sprachwissenschaft und Kommunikationsforschung, Band 14, Heft 4, 337, 1961.
61. Weigl, E.: The deblocking phenomenon of the speech function in aphasics. Proceedings of VII International Congress of Neurology, 1969.
62. Weinstein, E. & Kahn, R.: Denial of Illness. Charles C. Thomas, Springfield, Ill., 1955.
63. Wepman, J.: Recovery from Aphasia. Ronald Press, New York, 1951.
64. Wepman, J.: A conceptual model for the processes involved in recovery from aphasia. J Speech Hear Dis 18: 4, 1953.
65. Wepman, J.: Aphasia therapy: a new look. J Speech Hear Dis 37: 203, 1972.
66. Wepman, J.: Aphasia: language without thought or thought without language? ASHA 18: 131, 1976.
67. Wepman, J. & Morency, A.: Filmstrips as an adjunct to language therapy for aphasia. J Speech Hear Dis 28: 191, 1963.
68. Wiegel-Crump, C.: Agrammatism and aphasia. In: Y. Lebrun & R. Hoops (eds.), Recovery in Aphasics—Psycholinguistics 4, pp. 243–253. Swets & Zeitlinger, B.V., Amsterdam, 1976.
69. Wint, G.: The Third Killer. Abelard Schuman, New York, 1967.
70. Wulf, H.: Aphasia: My World Alone. Wayne State University Press, Detroit, 1973.

Part II

Selected Papers from the
World Federation of Neurology
Committee sessions

Part II

Selected Papers from the
Mental Retardation and Technology
committee session

Language recovery in aphasia from 3 to 6 months after stroke

IVAR REINVANG AND HARALD ENGVIK

Most studies on recovery from aphasia have focused on whether or not the patients improve and if treatment makes any significant contribution to the likelihood or magnitude of improvement. The general conclusion can be derived from these studies that excluding the first three months after stroke as a period in which spontaneous recovery is most likely to take place, a significant number of patients continue to improve in the further period from three to six months after stroke and even later. No definitive conclusions on the importance of treatment for this late recovery can be drawn on the basis of present data, but the work of Vignolo (7, 8) indicates that it is of importance.

One may argue that before further progress towards determining the efficacy of treatment can be made, two problems will have to be addressed. The first is how the contrast between treatment and no treatment shall be defined. The second is to decide what sort of parameters should be studied to reflect improvement. In connection with this last point it may also be argued that studies of pattern of recovery are imperative.

In studying the efficacy of treatment a distinction should be made between three conditions: Negative treatment, neutral treatment and positive treatment. Negative treatment is a condition in which the patient confronts people who do not properly understand the nature of his deficit and who therefore attempt to address or stimulate him in ways which he cannot grasp, and who expect him to perform in ways that are not consistent with his capability. The natural reaction of the patient is to withdraw from verbal interaction. Neutral treatment is a condition in which the nature of the patient's deficit is correctly appraised, so that he is addressed in a manner which makes him able to comprehend, and he is encouraged to make maximum use of intact verbal capabilities for communication. Positive treatment must be based on a correct appraisal of the patient's deficit. A plan is made for how to bring performances that are not within the patient's capability at the start of therapy within his capability. The rationale for selecting tasks for a therapy programme is not the communicative value of these tasks themselves, but their expected value in bridging the gap from performance at start of therapy and desired outcome.

In designing a study for comparing treatment with no treatment these three broad conditions should be kept separate. No scientific study should be necessary to prove that negative treatment is harmful in relation to the other two conditions. The only interesting problem is whether positive treatment is more efficacious than neutral treatment. This also means that studies comparing patient groups who have received some form of treatment with control groups of patients who have been discharged to their home without any follow-up or professional counseling of relatives, are in risk of proving the harmful effect of negative treatment rather than any effects of positive treatment.

The comparison group for a study on effect of therapy should then be a group of aphasics receiving neutral treatment in the sense defined above. This is not the same as stimulation therapy. Neutral treatment does not imply a shotgun approach, but a mode of relating to the patient based on specific knowledge of his defects in comprehension and production.

Describing the quality of change simply in terms of improved/not improved is clearly unsatisfactory. Granted that direction of change (positive or negative) is an important piece of information, describing type of change is equally imperative. Such a description should take into account that the language function is a composite function, a fact which is reflected in the numerous dimensions of aphasic impairment and corresponding to subtests of modern aphasia batteries. Not only scores on individual subtests, but profiles corresponding to characteristic configurations of performances (types of aphasia) must be noted. Finally the communicative aspect of language may not be properly characterized by quantitative scores on an aphasia battery, and some appraisal should be made of communicative ability independent of test scores. As a guideline for what kinds of results to expect in studies of pattern of recovery, the observation by Head (4) may be noted, stating that the characteristic patterns of deficit are usually retained in each individual case through recovery. On the other hand it is well known that patients often show a more global pattern of impairment in the acute stages of illness, and that characteristic types of aphasia may only be clearly discernible after this initial period (1). It is also a familiar observation that in the very mild aphasia patterns corresponding to Broca, Wernicke or anomic types can not be clearly distinguished.

Dividing the time span after injury in stroke patients into different ranges, one may distinguish between the initial period (0–2 months), the intermediate period (2–6 months) and the late recovery period (6 months and beyond). It is known that spontaneous recovery contributes significantly to recovery in the initial period, and that language recovery tends to follow a global course in many cases. As a foundation for the study of efficacy of language therapy in the intermediate period data is needed on the development under neutral treatment conditions (as defined above) of patients with serious enough aphasic disabilities that markedly different patterns of deficits can be distinguished. The present study aims to provide such data.

Methods

We use an aphasia examination based on the neurological model of aphasia as outlined by neurologists like Geschwind (2). The testing procedures associated with such a model have been worked out by Goodglass and Kaplan (3). Our procedure (5) follows similar lines but is somewhat shorter than the complete Boston diagnostic test. The test is comprised of the following parts: (A) Communication rating. The patient is asked questions about his occupation, interests, and leisure time activities. Performance is rated on a 0–4 rating scale. (B) On the basis of the same conversation the presence and severity of qualitative abnormalities like paraphasias, articulatory effort, hesitations, stereotypes and self corrections are noted. (C) The entire taperecorded conversation is transcribed, and the patient's answers to open ended questions is the basis for quantitative assessment of speech rate and utterance length. (D) The rest of the test consists of subtests measuring comprehension, repetition, naming, reading comprehension, oral reading and writing. See (5) for further details. On the basis of test results transformed into percentile scores, a decision is made whether the profile corresponds to a certain type of aphasia. Formalized decision rules are stated in appendix A.

Subjects

The group reported consists of all subjects in whom initial testing had been done between 2 and 6 months after injury with repeat of the test no sooner than one month later. The mean time after injury for the initial test was three months (range: 2–5 months), and for the retest 7.5 months (range: 3–30 months). Mean age is 52 years, range from 15 to 75 years. There were in all 33 patients, 22 of whom had suffered a vascular stroke. Another 8 had subdural or intracerebral hæmatomas caused by ruptured aneurysms or of unknown etiology.

There were two cases of trauma and one of encephalitis.

Treatment

All patients with aphasia admitted to Sunnaas Hospital undergo an initial period of testing, including both aphasia tests and additional psychological and sensory-motor tests. The results are communicated to physicians and therapists in the form of written or oral reports, usually within three weeks after admission. The patient is treated by a team of therapists consisting of occupational therapist, physical therapist and nurse. A speech therapist has recently joined the group, but the majority of the patients reported here have not received treatment by a speech therapist during their stay. There is no formally worked out programme of treatment, but the general guidelines stress the activation of relatively intact language abilities, and the importance of daily sessions. We conclude therefore that our treatment programme in the period here reported comes closest to satisfying the conditions of neutral treatment.

Results

Table I and II show the improvement of the patients on the aphasia test. In Table I the development recorded on rating scales is illustrated. There is signi-

Table I. *Improvement on rating scales*

Marked improvment ($p < 0.01$)	No improvement ($p > 0.05$)
Communication rating	Dysarthria
	Literal paraphasia
	Complex paraphasia
	Stereotypy
	Hesitations

ficant improvement in communicative ability. None of the other rating scales show a significant improvement. This indicates that if abnormal qualities of speech (paraphasia, stereotypes, hesitations etc.) are present to any marked degree in our patients, these traits seldomly improve.

Table II shows that with respect to comprehension the ability to perform spoken commands improves significantly, whereas the ability to point correctly to body parts or to comprehend ideas does not improve.

Most tests involving spoken responses show marked improvement. This is true both of tests of repetition, naming and oral reading. Comprehension of written material in the form of sentences improves significantly, whereas writing shows a moderate, but significant improvement. In order to avoid reporting ceiling effects as lack of improvement, follow-up results on tests in which the mean performance was less than one standard deviation below the maximum score have not been reported.

In Table III the classifications into types of aphasia at test and retest have been reported.

The main impression is that patterns of performances from test to retest are relatively stable, but in order to judge this, an examination of the individual test profiles has been carried out. On the basis of this scrutiny subjects were divided into three groups with respect to type of development. Judgements were based on performances on the comprehension, repetition and naming

Table II. *Improvement on subtests*

	Marked ($p < 0.01$)	Some ($0.05 < p < 0.01$)	None
Comprehension	Perform actions with objects and body parts	—	Ideas (yes/no). Body parts
Repetition	Words. Nonsense syllables	Sentences	—
Naming	Body parts and objects. Responsive. Object actions	Body actions	—
Oral reading	Letters. Words	—	—
Reading comp.	Sentences	—	Letters. Words
Writing	—	Writing	—

Table III. *Types of aphasia at test and retest*

Initial	Outcome
Global (7) ⟶	Global (3)
	Unclassifiable (2)
	Conduction (1)
	Broca (1)
Broca (7) ⟶	Broca (6)
	Unclassifiable (1)
Wernicke (1) ⟶	Wernicke (1)
Isolation syndrome (2) ⟶	Isolation syndrome (1)
	Broca (1)
Transcort. sens. (2) ⟶	Transcort. sens. (2)
Conduction (6) ⟶	Conduction (5)
	Unclassifiable (1)
Unclassifiable (8) ⟶	Unclassifiable (4)
	Broca (2)
	Wernicke (1)
	Isolation syndrome (1)

parts of the test. In addition to no improvement, global improvement corresponds to shift in all performances to a higher level on the scale, with retainment of the characteristic test profile obtained on first testing. Specific improvement implies that some performances develop out of proportion to others, thereby altering the profile of results.

An example of global improvement is given in Fig. 1.

In Figs. 2 and 3 an illustration is given of development in specific perfor-

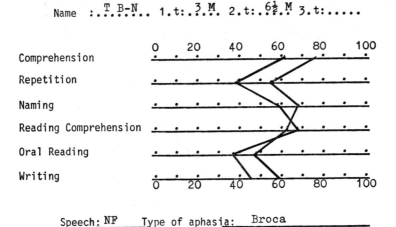

Name : T. B-N.. 1.t:.3.M. 2.t:.6½.M 3.t:.....

Speech: NF   Type of aphasia: Broca

Fig. 1. Global improvement.

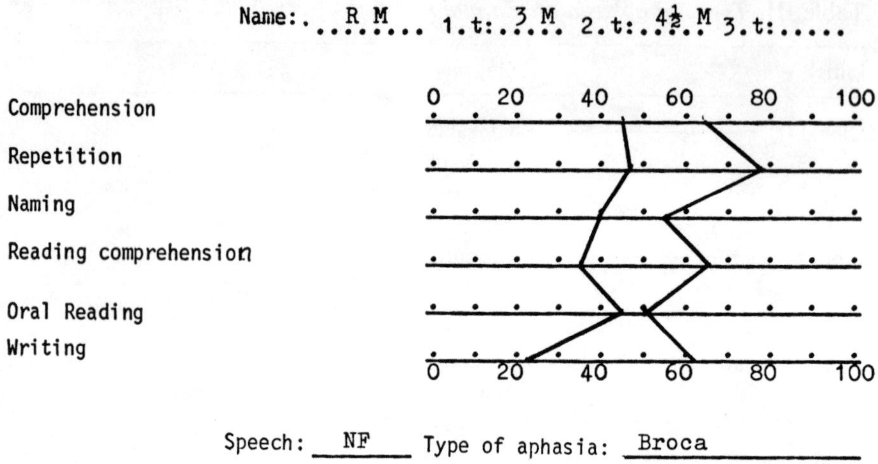

Name:. . . . . . . R M . . . 1.t:. . 3. M. . 2.t:. . 4½. M. 3.t:. . . . .

	0	20	40	60	80	100
Comprehension						
Repetition						
Naming						
Reading comprehension						
Oral Reading						
Writing	0	20	40	60	80	100

Speech: NF   Type of aphasia: Broca

Fig. 2. Specific improvement.

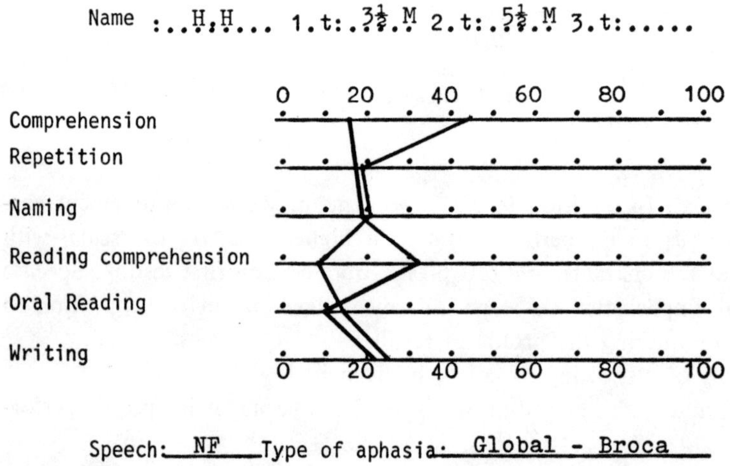

Name :. . H. H. . . 1.t:. 3½. M 2.t:. 5½. M 3.t:. . . . .

	0	20	40	60	80	100
Comprehension						
Repetition						
Naming						
Reading comprehension						
Oral Reading						
Writing	0	20	40	60	80	100

Speech: NF   Type of aphasia: Global - Broca

Fig. 3. Specific improvement.

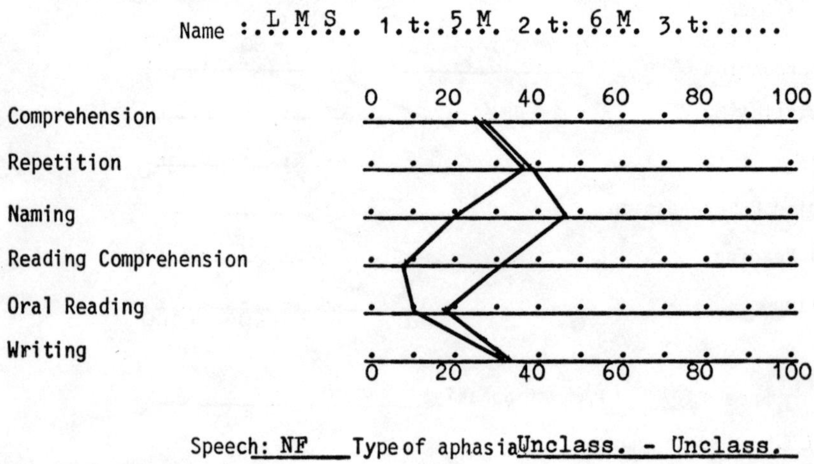

Name :. . L. M. S. . 1.t:. .5. M. 2.t:. .6. M. 3.t:. . . . .

	0	20	40	60	80	100
Comprehension						
Repetition						
Naming						
Reading Comprehension						
Oral Reading						
Writing	0	20	40	60	80	100

Speech: NF   Type of aphasia Unclass. - Unclass.

Fig. 4. Specific improvement.

Name : .. O B ... 1.t:. 5 M. 2.t:.. 7 M. 3.t:.....

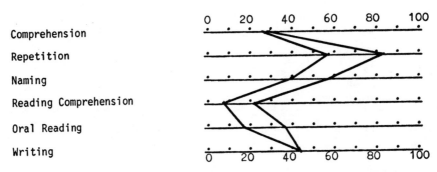

Speech: __NF__ Type of aphasia: Unclass. - Transcort. mot.

Fig. 5. Specific improvement.

Name: ..R.A... 1.t:3½.M. 2.t:.2½.år3.t:.....

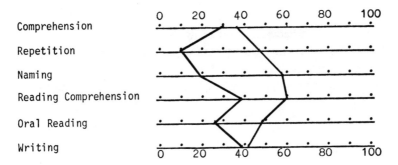

Speech: __NF__ Type of aphasia: Unclass. - Broca

Fig .6. Specific improvement.

Navn:. HMS .... 1.t:.. 4 .. 2.t:.. 12 .. 3.t:.....

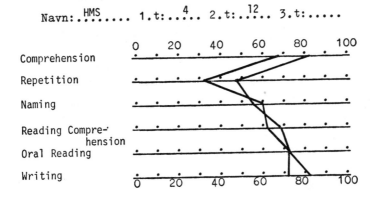

Speech: __F__ Type of aphasia : Conduction-Conduct.

Fig. 7. Specific improvement.

Table IV. *Type of development predicted by age and other variables*

	No improvement (N=7)	Global improvement (N=13)	Specific improvement (N=14)
Age (years)	58	48	50
Time after injury (months)	3.8	3.0	3.3
Test-retest interval (months)	2.5	3.0	6.0

Age: $F=0.978$, N.S. Time after injury: $F=1.157$, N.S. Test-retest interval: $F=1.776$, N.S.

mances related to comprehension or naming, with virtually no other improvements.

Finally more composite patterns are shown, classified as specific improvements, where repetition and naming develop jointly, but with little change in comprehension (Fig. 4), or improvement on comprehension and repetition takes place with no change in naming (Fig. 5).

A one way analysis of variance was performed to obtain evidence on differences in age, in time between onset of illness and initial testing, and in the interval between first and second testing between groups of patients showing different development patterns.

The results are shown in Table IV, where none of the obtained F-ratios are significant.

Discussion

The results show that improvement takes place to a significant degree in the time interval studied and under conditions that probably correspond to neutral treatment. The changes have been described across patients with respect to types of test performances and ratings showing most improvement. Changes have also been described within patients, with respect to the retainment or alteration of the characteristic performance profile obtained on first testing.

Changes across patients show most significant improvement on subtests involving oral language production and on rating of communicative ability. At initial testing the mean communication performance as rated by the examiner corresponds to a level where the patient is playing a passive role in communication, forcing the examiner continually to ask questions and formulate possible interpretations of what the patient may want to communicate. The rating at follow-up corresponds to a level at which the patient carries more of the burden of communication by supplying content material. There seems therefore to be a reasonable carryover of the improvement shown on formal testing into improvement of communication.

Comprehension of spoken language shows improvement only in the ability to carry out commands, but not of agnosic or conceptual disturbances. The results on reading comprehension with marked improvement on comprehension of sentences and no improvement on letters or words, probably indicates that on first testing most patients are able to comprehend letters and words, but not sentences. At follow-up those severely alexic subjects who did not comprehend letters and words on first testing have progressed little. Those patients having problems mainly with comprehending sentences, have probably been able to partly overcome their problem on the basis of their skill in reading letters and words.

There is only moderate recovery of ability to write, and it is the author's impression that when such recovery takes place it comes relatively late in development.

Looking at changes within patients, the classification into types of aphasia at initial testing and follow-up seems on the whole to confirm Head's opinion that characteristic profiles are retained. When another method of classification, based on a visual impression of relationships between scaled scores is employed, this conclusion is less obvious. Of the patients who show improvement, about half show a pattern of global improvement, and the rest show a pattern of specific improvement. It would be tempting to hypothesize that such patterns correspond to developments in the early as opposed to the late part of the period under discussion, but such an hypothesis does not receive support from our statistical analyses.

It seems then that our results may contribute to a better description of patterns of recovery, which was our aim. The problems of predicting different patterns of recovery have been approached in a previous study from our laboratory (6) and will be more fully discussed in a subsequent paper.

Appendix. Rules for classifying types of aphasia on the basis of test profiles

Speech is classified as fluent, non-fluent, mixed or normal.

Fluent: Words per min (WPM) > 80, utterance length (UL) > 5.0, speech quality abnormal.

Non-fluent: WPM < 50, UL < 4.0. In terms of ordering on a percentile scale, non-fluent corresponds to the low end of the scale.

Mixed: Abnormal quality of speech, neither fluent nor non-fluent.

1. Severe aphasias.

Global aphasia. Non-fluent speech. Scores within the bottom 20 percentile points on comprehension, repetition and naming. If the 20th percentile corresponds to raw score of zero, the cut off point is adjusted to the score at 20 percentile points above raw score of zero.

Jargon aphasia. Fluent speech. Scores on comprehension, repetition and naming as in global aphasia.

2. Aphasias with large differences between performance on comprehension, repetition and naming. (Large difference means difference of at least 20 percentile points.)

Isolation syndrome. Non-fluent speech. Repetition better than naming. Repetition better than comprehension.

Transcortical sensory aphasia. Fluent speech. Repetition better than naming. Repetition better than comprehension.

Conduction aphasia. Fluent or mixed speech. Comprehension better than repetition.

Anomic aphasia. Fluent speech. Comprehension better than naming. Repetition better than naming.

3. Aphasias with more homogeneous performances.

Broca's aphasia. Non-fluent speech. Comprehension better than fluency. Naming better than fluency.

Wernicke's aphasia. Fluent speech. Comprehension worse than fluency. Repetition worse than fluency.

4. Slight aphasia. Scores within top ten percentile points on comprehension, repetition and naming.

Given an individual profile the applicability of type designations is tested in the order listed. The search stops when an applicable designation has been found.

References

1. Benson, D. F. & Geschwind, N.: The Aphasias. In: A. B. Baker (ed.), Handbook of Clinical Neurology. Vol. 1. Harper and Row, New York, 1974.
2. Geschwind, N.: The organization of language and the brain. Science 170: 940, 1970.
3. Goodglass, H. & Kaplan, E.: The Assessment of Aphasia. Lea and Febiger, Philadelphia, 1972.
4. Head, H.: Aphasia and Kindred Disorders of Speech. Macmillan, New York, 1926.
5. Reinvang, I. & Graves, R.: A basic aphasia examination. Scand J Rehab Med 7: 129, 1975.
6. Reinvang, I., Hjeltnes, N. & Guvaag, S. P.: Afasibehandling av hjerneslagpasienter. T Norske Lægeforening 27: 1421, 1976.
7. Vignolo, L. A.: Evaluation of aphasia and language rehabilitation: Retrospective exploratory study. Cortex 1: 344, 1964.
8. Vignolo, L. A.: The effect of language rehabilitation in the outcome of aphasia. Paper presented at International Neuropsychology Society Conference, Oxford, England, Aug. 1, 1977.

Family treatment in aphasia— experience from a patient association

STINA LINELL AND GÖRAN STEG

Introduction

Aphasia produces many social and psychological problems and it is, there-fore, important that family members cooperate in the treatment of aphasic patients. After the initial period of hospital treatment the responsibility for the patient is shifted to the family. There is a strong need for continuing help for the patient and his family after discharge which must be met by organiza-tions other than those purely medical. There is a need for a patient associa-tion for aphasic patients and their families. Such an association should have certain objectives:

To increase knowledge of the syndromes of aphasia amongst patients and relatives as well as in society as a whole.

To work for increased contact between members of the association through meetings, excursions, clubs, and studygroups etc.

To support research in the field.

To work for better resources in society and within the hospital system for the rehabilitation of patients with aphasia.

With these aims a patient association for aphasia was founded in Gothenburg in the beginning of 1976. Similar organizations have been started in Stockholm in 1974, in Malmö 1976 and in Uppsala 1977.

Members belong to three categories: Persons with aphasia, their relatives, and other interested persons including the medical staffs of rehabilitation and neurological clinics etc. The association is supported financially through membership fees and grants from individuals, funds, and official organizations.

The number of members is steadily increasing and has now reached around 1,000 persons in the different organizations taken together. A national organization is planned and will be started. Hopefully, the national organiza-tion will inform and influence the authorities in questions concerning clinical problems of aphasia and the development of aphasia rehabilitation facilities. It should also encourage the training of speech therapists. The board of the national organization will have representatives for both patients, their relatives, and the medical staffs concerned with treatment. A balance is essential between patient's representatives and medical experts in order to promote realistic policies for the organization.

The association has existed for less than two years and therefore follow-up results are not available. The following description presents the current activities of the association. It refers to the programme sent out twice a year presenting the different activities.

Information on aphasia

Lectures on the nature of aphasia and rehabilitation are given twice a year in small groups not exceeding 15 participants, four evenings once a week. First a physician provides basic information on the nature of aphasia, secondly a speech pathologist describes the different therapeutic methods. A third lecture is a collaborative discussion by the team of physician, speech pathologist, occupational therapist, social worker, psychologist, physiotherapist, and nurse. A fourth lecture on family therapy is given by a psychologist. This form of lectures permits close contact and realistic discussion among the persons with aphasia, their relatives (including their children) and the medical staff. It has proved to be very valuable.

A written folder providing information on the nature of aphasia and the patient organization has been distributed to hospitals, social authorities, police, taxi drivers, and others.

A personal information card to be carried by patients describes their special handicap and is intended to be used by the patient in situations where communication is difficult.

Social and group activities

After discharge from hospital and after the termination of systematic aphasia treatment, group activities within the patient organizations are initiated. The aim of the group activities is to activate speech and thought. Groups of 8–10 patients read and discuss books. This activity is complemented by visits to museums. Between 40 and 50 members of the society in Gothenburg regularly take part in these group activities.

Once a month a social event is scheduled in which 70–80 members of the association participate. The program usually includes a lecture, entertainment, and refreshments. On these occasions members have the opportunity to meet each other and also to meet members of the medical staff. The lectures have been devoted to problems of aphasia, language, brain function, and therapeutic methods i.e. music therapy, family therapy. The facilities available in the society for handicapped people have also been described.

A conversation group, an art club, and lectures on ceramics are available for members. Other groups are studying English, taking part in "rhythmical activation" or participating in different handicrafts.

The association keeps inexpensive theatre tickets available for members and excursions are arranged with participation of all family members. Often the patients' children take an active part in the activities.

In cooperation with the hospital library and the communal libraries a library service has been organized for association members. Tape recorders and tapes with appropriate texts are also available.

A steadily growing number of members have made use of the opportunities offered by the patient organization. This fact makes it appear that the association is always concerned with identifying the realistic needs of its members and attempting to meet them.

The society has taken part in negotiations with the University authorities regarding the development of a speech pathology training program. Plans have been advanced for a training program of logopeds and speech therapists in Gothenburg in connection with the Rehabilitation, Neurological and Otological clinics. When this academic program begins basic resources for aphasia research will be available in Gothenburg.

It is apparent that a patient organization of this kind serves the needs of a group of patients who are seriously handicapped and left without adequate supportive services after hospitalization.

Broca's aphasia: what is to be re-trained?

O. SABOURAUD, J. GAGNEPAIN, A. DUVAL AND H. GUYARD

The question raised in this paper proceeds from the opinion that both the methods for re-education and the results are unsatisfactory in the field of Broca's aphasia (10,3). According to a prevailing opinion, this group of aphasias should be considered as "aphasia *plus*", i.e., either aphasia *plus* dysarthria or aphasia *plus* inhibition.

For years we have pursued another line of research (12). Its main theme is that Broca's aphasia and Wernicke's aphasia designate two fundamentally different types of disturbances. If this is so, the study of the specific disturbance underlying Broca's aphasia should be the first step towards a better approach to the rehabilitation of these patients.

This paper deals with two topics:

1. The nature of the aphasic disturbances in the "Broca" group.
2. The role of dysarthria and inhibition and the relation of these two disorders to the aphasic disturbance (as well as to other cortical syndromes).

As soon as the specificity of Broca's aphasia is no longer ascribed to the mere presence of dysarthria and (or) inhibition, one must indicate the criteria for inclusion of aphasic patients in the group. It seems to us that the most viable rule to form groups among the population of aphasics is to unify the symptoms which are usually observed together and the clinical pictures which follow one another as evolution proceeds (progression or regression). According to this rule, a group may be recognized, whose most severe picture consists of stereotyped utterances, whose main aspects are defined as agrammatism on the one hand and reduction of contrasts in the phonic chain on the other hand. This group can easily be contrasted to Wernicke's aphasia, a group including the evolutions from jargon to paraphasias of either verbal or phonemic nature.

I. THE NATURE OF THE APHASIC DISTURBANCES

We can start by defining language as a cultural system, the function of which is to mediate human representation. This system results from the interplay of elements—the linguistic signs—whose definition proceeds exclusively from their reciprocal relations inside the system, and not from the external world. The inclusion of signs within a system differentiate them from mere symbols:

the symbolic relation is dual (between symbolizing and symbolized thing), while the linguistic system introduces the relation between analysed sound (becoming "Signifiant" = Signifier) and analysed sense (becoming "Signifié" = Signified).

Following these few definitions, aphasic troubles can be said to disrupt the functioning of the linguistic system i.e. the functioning of an analysis of sense (the analysis which gives rise to the field of *Signifié*), and of an analysis of sound (the analysis which supports the existence of *Signifiant*).

Aphasic disturbances can interfere either on the level of *Signifié* or on the level of *Signifiant*, both types of disturbance commonly being present to a greater or lesser extent in the same patient.

The main contribution of aphasiology to the knowledge of language is, in our opinion, that analysis, i.e. the functioning of a cultural system, is not a simple but a double process, and double on the level of *Signifié*, as well as on the level of *Signifiant*. There is not one kind of aphasia, but two.

Each kind of aphasia may be considered as the break-down of one capacity, the conjunction of the two capacities being equally essential to the functioning of the analysis (on the level of *Signifié*, as well as on the level of *Signifiant*). With this background, Broca's aphasia appears to be the disruption of a generative capacity (while Wernicke's aphasia concerns a taxonomic capacity). Through the study of Broca's aphasia, we shall discover how such a generative capacity intervenes in the working up of the linguistic system. The kind of approach we are discussing is reminiscent to some degree of the differentiation by Jakobson (6, 7) among aphasic symptoms of a syntagmatic and a para-digmatic disorder. This concept of a double nature of aphasia, after having raised much interest, has been abandoned by most aphasiologists, in favour of a unitary and linear conception of language, described as a series of opera-tions from thought to speech. We maintain that, with an appropriate develop-ment of the theory of language, the dichotomy between generative and taxonomic capacities working in conjunction, and hence of two main groups of aphasias, is an aid to the disclosure of new facts.

The conception that Broca's aphasia represents a selective impairment of a generative capacity (leading to the ruin of the whole linguistic analysis), will be discussed successively on the level of *Signifié* and on the level of *Signifiant*.

The question of stereotyped utterances will appear more understandable at the end of the discussion.

A. *The level of signifié (signified)*

On this level, the clinical picture characteristic of Broca's aphasia is what is generally called agrammatism, This disturbance is diagnosed with no great difficulty in such simple examples as:

— monsieur, valise, marcher (gentleman, suit-case, walk)
— un garçon, i'joue, trois, trois billes (a boy, he plays, three, three balls).

Incidentally, agrammatism is easier to recognize than to strictly define, being restricted neither to the absence of the article, nor to the infinitive form of verbs, nor to the lack of prepositions, etc. ... (on this resistance to definition, see Tissot et al. (14)).

This difficulty clearly shows that neurology has nothing to expect from the use of such entities as what classical grammarians call "words". The conception of a process underlying formal categories and revealing the activity of this or that particular capacity will prove to be much more promising. Along these lines we shall discuss the following points:

1) that agrammatism represents the lack of a generative capacity,
2) contrasting with the preservation of a taxonomic capacity.

These two formulas are not sufficient to account for the whole of the observations of Broca's aphasia; they need to be completed by the following:

3) there is a loss of morphology
4) leading to a peculiar and abnormal usage of syntax.

1. The lack of a generative capacity

That Broca's aphasia is a deficit, appears evident in such an example as:

Tell us about your journey—"Lourdes" (a pilgrimage)
What did you do? "prié" (prayed),

where the patient's expression is reduced to a unitary designation, and nothing is added to it.

A very similar example: "Jean-Yves, Thérèse, foin, tracteur" (J.Y., Th., hay, tractor) a sequence appearing as a succession of designations, with no link between the items as indicated by linguistic marks, the linkage being in the things, not in the text.

The same kind of deficit is also found in this expression: "Sylvain et Sylvette, ils entendent, Sylvain et Sylvette, ils ont peur, Sylvain et Sylvette, ils partent, etc." (S. and S., they hear, S. and S. they are afraid, S. and S., they get away).

Here the term "agrammatism" does not strictly apply, as long as we find articles and conjugation of verbs; nevertheless the successivity of unitary designations is the same and justifies grouping these different aspects together under a common heading, which we propose to call a reduction of textual contrasts.

2. The fitness of taxonomy is intact

This formulation recalls a very old observation: that agrammatic patients, while uttering infrequently a word, with little or no variety of contrasts along the text, make use of the most exact terms, the most informative, and eventually of uncommon words if exactness and information require them.

They seemingly rely on this intact capacity in order to compensate the lacking one.

Such an impression of precise and informative choices can be considered as the preference given by the patients to "words" which have nothing in common one to the other, which belong to independent semantic fields.

This remark will become understandable when we are aware of the difficulties encountered by aphasic patients in introducing new and different elements through linguistic matrices; it is no surprise then if they compensate through non-linguistic relations, and increase the distance between the terms they produce. Among three terms, they choose the two more remote and neglect the nearest; such a distance of course is relative to situation, since, e.g., sheep and pig are near compared to elephant, but remote compared to ewe, and quite independent of any formalisation by a linguistic system.

In any case, as soon as we recognize the precision of agrammatic choices, we are compelled to remark that this correctness is somewhat limited and surprisingly subject to "mistakes"; quite commonly, an agrammatic patient gives "buy" in place of "sell", reads "school" for "pupil", and is not disturbed by a sentence such as "the mouse catches the cat". All these examples show that the "mistakes" are not just chance replacements. They bring forth the idea that the linguistic frame of one word unites a plurality of lexical items (i.e. the products of taxonomic operations, which we call "Semes"). In the last examples, some of the "Semes" were correct, and some were, apparently, neglected, the most neglected being those Semes that refer to the relations internal to a text supposed to be organized as a whole. This new insight onto the Word as a pattern of organization for several Semes introduces the next point.

3. The loss of accidence

In a first step, lack of generative capacity has appeared as a difficulty in building up a whole out of elements. No less important is the concurrent difficulty to disrupt a whole into constitutive units. (How did you come?) "by car", gives the patient no facility to name the toy car presented on the table. The de-construction is as impaired as the building up; the lack of generative capacity results in the loss of a basic unit along the axis of text, which is the Word (as a linguistic entity.)

The loss of the unit: Word enlightens many aspects of Broca's aphasia. First, the patient tends to produce on several substrates several semes which are normally unified through the use of one word, a symptom which we call diffraction. E.g. a patient should write "woman waiter" for "waitress" (Transposition of a french example: "dame coiffeur" for "coiffeuse").

Then, the loss of the Word as a unit makes it understandable to observe frequent misuses of word-types, e.g. nouns and verbs as different patterns of organization for semes. The undifferentiation may be absolute, the patient

producing only lexemes, in the so-called telegraphic style: "enfants, manger ..."
(children, eat).

In a less complete form, one may find either noun or verb indicators, but quite haphazardly: "D'autres viennent et les donner l'argent" (others come and the give the money).

More often the fundamental difference between Noun and Verb is present, but in a fixed, unique, manner. "Les enfants, *je* bois (the children, *I* drink). Elle dit à sa maman ... Jérome ... *Je* peux manger ... avec nous", (she says, to her mother, Jerome ... *I* can eat ... whith us"). The article then indicates the noun, the pronoun "I" indicates the verb. There remains nothing like a nominal pattern consisting of simultaneous choices of an "article" (the, a, some, etc.) together with a "preposition" (with, on, in, under, etc.), notwithstanding derivational suffixes (Isle, Islet), — vs. a verbal pattern the choices of which are between "I, you, he, she ..." preceded or not by "because, that, while, ..." including proper suffixes of conjugation. In the situation of aphasia, a functioning pattern seems to be replaced by a material form.

The use of material milestones instead of patterns of organization accounts for a kind of redundancy most common during rehabilitation, and for perseveration of models of sentences, leading eventually to nonsense. "Les enfants ils chantent, ... Maman, ala dit, Papa, ala rigole ..." (the children, they sing, ... Mamma, s'he says, Daddy s'he laughs). (What is a fisherman?) "c'est un homme qui pêche ..." (he's a man who goes fishing) (What is a tractor?) "c'est un homme qui conduit" (he's a man who goes driving). It does not seem justified to separate two kinds of agrammatism (as proposed by Tissot et al.) according to the presence or absence of these particular disturbances. The loss of Word as a unit essentially implies an impairment of any morphological achievement... In fact, the evolution appears continuous in the same patients from the lack of accidence to the inappropriate use of noun or verb indicators, etc. Here the advantage is clear of referring to capacity and processes, instead of such things as prepositions or pronouns.

4. Syntagmatic influence without true syntax

A syntagm may be defined as a pool of words within a text, recognizable on this mark that they possess at least one seme in common: once a taxonomic choice is made, it remains for the whole group (e.g. the sharing of plural by several words). The preceding development on the loss of the basic unit of text makes it clear that, whatever may be the persistence of any sense in common from one element to other elements uttered in one sequence, this persistence cannot establish a true syntagm, since it does not mark the crossing of boundaries between nonexisting Words. It means only repetition or perseveration. Only the ability of contrasting one to the other consecutive units gives purpose to the eventual sharing of one identity by two or more units. The examples given above of diffraction and of redundancy show that aphasic patients may maintain one taxonomic choice made once as a mere material substrate to introduce any new taxonomic element.

The difficulty for such patients seems precisely to make use of their taxonomic abilities and to produce new semes, notwithstanding the lack of word organization.

It must be realized that one basic result of the functioning system of language is the constant renewal of expressions. When analysis fails either in Broca's or in Wernicke's aphasia, perseveration occurs. Taxonomy is necessary for generativity to work properly, just as much as generativity (supposed to be lacking in Broca's aphasia) is for taxonomic achievements. But, perseveration manifests itself in a different manner according to the nature of the deficit: in Broca's aphasia it is reminiscent of the normal and purposeful persistence of semes in the course of the text; in Wernicke's aphasia, it looks like an adhesiveness to one seme as a false paradigmatic relation without true paradigm.

The difficulty of avoiding repetition in Broca's aphasia may at the very end account for the occurrence of stereotypy.

B. *The level of "signifiant" (signifier)*

The impact of Broca's aphasia on phonology (i.e. on the analysis of sound which gives rise to *Signifiant*) may be isolated or it may be associated to agrammatism and, if so, phonological disturbance may be dominant or accessory.

This assertion implies:

(a) that there exists a phonological disturbance, different from a motor trouble of speech articulation,
(b) that the disorder on the level of *Signifiant* is not identical in Broca's and in Wernicke's aphasia.

To account for the phonological disturbance in Broca's aphasia it appears advantageous to follow the same steps as for the level of *Signifié*:

1) there is a lack of generative capacity
2) while taxonomy is spared
3) The unit or phoneme is not available as a bundle of distinctive features,
4) excessive perseveration replaces significative duplication.

1. The tendency to reproduce several times one and the same "phoneme" along one sequence, with the variants of anticipation, perseveration, simplification of clusters, is by itself a deficit in the building-up of a whole out of multiple elements.

    Examples: "ku ke" for: "couper" kupe (To cut), "tri' trã" for: "trident" (tridã) "bi' bi' to' tet'" for "bibliothèque" (library). We propose that all these deficiencies be grouped under the common heading of a reduction of contrasts along the phonic chain.

2. If this semi-quantitative reduction is obvious, the elements actually produced appear quite in agreement with the expected model. And this relative conformity would not make it unreasonable to speak of a sparing of taxonomic choice between distinctive features. This notion is relatively reinforced, when one observes a patient trying through successive attempts, to complete the model but failing because the production of a new correct feature cannot occur without the loss of another properly given before.

Ex: "structure" (Stryktyr) → trys'tyr, strys'tyr, tryk'tyr. But even by combining these two principles—deficit in the building up of a whole, sparing of correct choice—one could not expect to cover the field of the actual production by patients. Very often indeed proper sounds are introduced but in the wrong place so much so that not only are whole phonemes exchanged (pu–ke for Ku pe, couper = to cut) but sometimes one or two distinctive features in each phoneme of a pair: "ku–de" for: "goûter" (gute). A phoneme appears then as the grouping and the organization of multiple features into one unit. A difficulty in dealing with patterns necessary to bring features together, appears in instances like: "skres" for: "trèfle" (shamrock).

Distinctive features can be considered as the basic elements for taxonomic choice, while the phoneme constitutes the unit for generative performance.

3. The lack of generative capacity appears to be at the same time a trouble in building up a phonic chain, as well as in taking a whole into constitutive pieces. The unit called phoneme just results from generative capacity. The lack of this unit appears to account for many aspects of Broca's aphasia.

The cutting of the speech continuum into syllabic utterances is common in aphasic productions. It is by no means specific, being also a possible result of dysarthria or dyspneumia. But the utterance of any new syllable is utilised by aphasics as a substrate to introduce every new feature. "Xavier" (Ksavje)— "Za' Vje ... Kiz' ... Za' Vje ... Kar' Zje ... za' za' Ksa' zje" Diffraction is also a phenomenon of the phonological level: "ga' Ka' Sa' Vje".

The syllable appears then as the basic performance of sound articulation, and not as a combination of phonemes: it is utilized by aphasics as a substitute for the missing linguistic unit. The phoneme on the contrary may be conceived as a pattern of feature organization, as a unit necessary to build up and also to take into pieces phonic chains. The lack of these functions clarifies the observation of aphasic utterances.

A loss of the basic unit apparently makes it difficult to introduce new contrasts in a chain of sounds, leading to many kinds of perseveration. Perseveration makes no sense, contrasting with normal purposeful duplication which is characteristic of some words.

Most common and typical in Broca's aphasia is the perseveration of a type of syllable:

coquelicot (ko kli ko) — "klokliklo ... kokliklo"
It may be more severe as in: "bi" bi' to' tet'" (bibliothèque)

One step more and a word will be reproduced "en-bloc" in order to designate different objects: this type of perseveration may occur when the examiner adds a third object to two already present, or even, when the second one is placed along the first.

Thus the very same disturbance may be found to occur on different scales, "words" or syllables and culminates in stereotyped utterances. Perseveration is by no means a unique characteristic of Broca's aphasia. In Wernicke's aphasia also, at the level of *Signifiant*, the lack of taxonomic capacity leads to a kind of perseveration in consecutive attempts. It may be either jargon: "anafade, anašézatide"; or paraphasia: "grir, ŭ grir ro, ŭ grore, ŭ p'ti grelo, grodile, grəle ..." (attempts to name: a small bell, called: un grelot). In these instances patients proceed just as we do when we decline the cases of a word, but for the fact that what they organize are no more semes nor distinctive features. One capacity is necessary for the efficiency of the other; the lack of one leads the other to the situation of perseveration. But depending upon the nature of the deficit (generative or taxonomic), the type of perseveration looks quite different.

This difference has been suspected by many observers who have tried to demonstrate the reality of it (4, 5, 8). Unfortunately these attempts proved to be unsuccessful, and the authors were forced to the conclusion that there was only one disturbance as far as phonological analysis is concerned. This failure, supported the proponents of a unique "phonetic encoding" procedure, making the difference between Broca's and Wernicke's aphasias the presence or absence of an associated dysarthric disturbance.

We can bring a new argument to the debate. All the attempts to study the phonic chains produced by aphasics refer the actual product to the expected chain, then record the mistakes, and compare one mistaken phoneme to the correct one, either in terms of similarity, or in terms of contiguity if not in terms of logical transformations. With this method of recording "mistakes", the observer introduces his own cutting out and his own units and he is compelled to consider the pathologic product as if the choice among these units had been deficient or disturbed. At the same time, he takes it for granted that pertinence is always dependable and he focuses his approach on acoustic or articulatory phenomena for the reason that linguistic criteria are missing.

We have designed another method of testing, which is effective as soon as patient can (after demonstration) give the name of three objects. We utilize triads of homeophones:

— "écran, écrin, écrou" (ekrã, ekrẽ ekru = screen, case, screw)
— chapeau, chateau, chameau" (šapo, šato, šamo = hat, castle, camel)

The examiner shows successively two pictures, until the naming is correct or stable; then he shows another pair; all three items are paired the same way and each pair presented in reverse order.

The overall result is that, with Broca's aphasics, displacements of phonemes far from being fortuitous do follow a rule; if we take into account that in every triad one pair of homeophones is less "distant" than the other two (ekrã–ekrẽ are nearer to each other than ekrã–ekru or ekrẽ–ekru). We observe that the greater distance regularly contaminates the shorter one, the latter being unstable and frequently the locus of errors.

In contrast the mistakes of Wernicke's aphasics do not borrow elements only from the actual test situation and they follow no rule at all. The results of this study, which is still in progress, seem to establish the reality of a difference between two types of phonological deficits. It directly derives from the conception of a loss of phoneme in Broca's aphasia, a lack of distinctiveness in Wernicke's aphasia.

One possible consequence of this last research is to make understandable why observers believe at first sight that Broca's aphasics replace voiced by unvoiced phonemes and why recording data about actual mistakes discards this hypothesis. In fact, when they speak, these patients contaminate in any phonological sequence short-distance pairs of sounds and favour long-distance pairs: e.g. in the word "bibliothèque" (bi) (bli), and (t) (k) are short distance and vanish in presence of (b) (t) or (b) (k): this gives: bi' bi' to' tet'.

Depending upon a particular chain, this alteration may give the impression that the number of unvoiced, highly contrasted phonemes is increased, while the number of individual exchanges from unvoiced to voiced is actually balanced by the reverse replacements.

II. THE STATUS OF INHIBITION AND DYSARTHRIA

One advantage of defining Broca's aphasia in terms of linguistic criteria is to be able to diagnose it apart from inhibition and dysarthria. Nevertheless even if the latter troubles are neither the most frequent, nor the most important in many cases, they ought to be discussed, as they influence the prognosis and interfere with rehabilitation.

A. *Inhibition*

This behavioral and descriptive parameter is commonly mentioned by speech-therapists in order to express the difficulty they encounter in making the Broca's patient say one word, or answer with more than rare and brief utterances to their own verbal display.

The term, inhibition, refers to neuro-physiology, but brings to mind, when applied to aphasics, the clinical pictures sometimes observed after frontal lesions.

Luria has particularly stressed the role of the frontal lobes as regulators of behavior. Following this author, we can consider two types of inhibition as frequently observed in case of frontal lesions:

(a) An inhibition of all pragmatic performances (accompanied or not by excess of affective and instinctive output) with underactivity, latency, lack of a personal production as added to the pre-existing situation.

(b) A specialized type of inhibition, which concerns only speech activity, and is described by LURIA under the name of "dynamic aphasia". Even if "aphasia" is perhaps not the best name for a behavioral anomaly which spares linguistic analysis, the reality of this clinical picture is beyond doubt: rare utterances (but grammatically correct) frequently limited to "yes", or "no", lack of initiative, lack of personal production, patient's tendency to incorporate in the answer the very terms of the question.

This "dynamic aphasia" seems to occur after some frontal lesions, predominantly left frontal, sparing the cortical areas essential for language. It seems important to point out that such an inhibition involving speech initiative and behavior acts in the same direction as the aphasic disorders in generative capacity: repetition, difficulty in introducing new and different elements.

Perhaps, at the same time, one should recall that there exists some kind of behavioral syntax in the monitoring of action (see LASHLEY) which is especially dependent on the functioning of the frontal lobes in primates. But it goes without saying that the generative capacity, insofar as it is engaged in a linguistic analysis, acquires a completely new status through the projection onto and the dependence upon taxonomic capacity.

B. *Dysarthria*

This neurological category has long been considered as the distinctive symptom of Broca's aphasia, although it is not necessarily present, at least to the mind of neurologists who accept that inhibitory factors do not involve solely speech articulation, and that impairment in the production of a phonic chain may be an aphasic disorder affecting the linguistic analysis of sound (the "*Signifiant*" face of the linguistic sign).

Moreover, dysarthria as a disorder possibly associated with aphasia is not strictly defined. It has been isolated as a cortical dysarthria, different from myopathic, bulbar, pseudo-bulbar, cerebellar, striatal ... dysarthrias. This negative status is not sufficient as the description of cortical dysarthria soon reveals that it is not a unique, but a multiple syndrome. Alajouanine et al. (1) have distinguished three kinds of "anarthria": paretic, dystonic and dyspraxic. By means of clinical and oscillographic criteria, (13) we have been able to recognize two and probably three types of cortical dysarthrias; the comparison with pseudo-bulbar, cerebellar and parkinsonian dysarthrias does not lead to an interpretation of these types of cortical dysarthrias as paretic or dystonic and suggests another basis for explanation.

(a) We have observed exclusively in connection with Broca's aphasia a first type of dysarthria, characterized by the reduction of sound utterances to a preferential scheme, e.g. occlusive or (h) at the beginning of the first syllable, l, m, or n, at the beginning of the second one. There may be minimal variations, the essential uniformity of performance being maintained all the time.

Dysarthric patients of this kind are different from those whose trouble is only phonological with such productions as: "bi' bi' to' tet'" or "krys kyr" because they tend to introduce minimal sound differences through their uniform performance: "ato", for (bateau = ship) "ta' tan'" for (gendarme = policeman), "'oten" for (hôtel).

It must be said that this type of cortical dysarthria is not completely unrelated to the lack of generative capacity which is present in Broca's aphasia. Both result in a tendency to repeat one and the same production, so that both aphasic troubles and dysarthria may contribute to the genesis of stereotypy.

The preferential scheme is also reminiscent of the behavior studied by Luria after lesions of the premotor regions of the frontal lobes. This premotor syndrome is demonstrable as well in gestures (the fist-ring test) in drawings (the square, triangle, cross, circle series), in rhythm reproductions; in all kinds of performances, it presents itself as a tendency to reproduce a uniform, badly-differentiated pattern, and to obliterate the contrasts in any sequence. At the same time, premotor patients are unable to program a complex task by cutting it out into successive steps.

From this comparison, it can be considered that there may be a physiological function related to building programs of action and differentiating successive performances—that this function may be disturbed in the field of speech articulation (dysarthria)—and that generative capacity proceeds from this same function, but for the fact it is engaged in the process of mediation through the analysis of a cultural system.

(b) Another type of cortical dysarthria should be mentioned because it is, in our experience, far more frequent than the preceding one. This second type is composed of two audible anomalies (visible on the oscillogram):

— presence of multiple superimposed noises before the production of consonants,
— ample variations during the emission of a single wowel (or voiced phoneme), so that it appears as a succession of different phonemes on the oscillogram, and it is heard as a diphthong (this is specially noticeable in French, where diphthongs have no place in the system).

We suggest comparison of this dysarthria to the hand performance in so-called ideomotor dyspraxia: the hand lacks clear direction, cannot be inserted on the proper substrate, cannot be oriented in the correct plane.

The dysarthric type under discussion has been observed in our experience in connection with Broca's and Wernicke's aphasia and a few times as an independent disorder.

(c) There may be a third type of dysarthria which we have observed in connection with Wernicke's aphasia in two cases of our series. It presents itself as a kind of very fast stuttering, which on the oscillogram appears as pseudo-phonetic attempts, preceding the production of jargon, or paraphasias, or even some normal words.

If confirmed on a larger scale, this third type could be considered as a difficulty in selecting the right motor performance, thus indicating that the taxonomic capacity, basic for language analysis, derives also from a physiological parameter.

We shall *summarize* the preceding considerations on inhibition and dysarthria by saying that if an approach to the aphasias as a disturbance of capacities (and not as a loss of words) can easily be harmonized with a theory of language as a cultural mediation, it is not incompatible at the same time with a physiology of the brain, each capacity being not linguistic by itself but as a result of their mutual interplay.

As a *conclusion*, we may ask a question about the method followed during this research: is it clinical observation? or theoretical discussion? We should like to bring the two questions into one, as isolated observation would only rely on categories of grammatical teaching, and theory alone has no other importance than to force a new questioning of known facts.

References

1. Alajouanine, Th., Ombredane, A. & Durand, M.: Le syndrome de désintégration phonétique dans l'aphasie. 1 vol. Masson, Paris, 1939.
2. Alajouanine, Th., Lhermitte, F., Ledoux, Renaud, P. & Vignolo, L. A.: Les composantes phonémiques et sémantiques de la jargonaphasie. Rev Neurol 110/1: 5, 1964.
3. Basso, A., Faglioni, P. & Vignolo, L. A.: Etude contrôlée de la rééducation du langage dans l'aphasie: comparaison entre aphasiques traités et non traités. Rev Neurol 131: 607, 1975.
4. Blumstein, Sh. E.: Some phonological implications of aphasic speech. In: Psycholinguistics and aphasia. 1 vol. The Johns Hopkins University Press, Baltimore, 1973.
5. Blumstein, Sh. E.: A phonological investigation of aphasic speech. 1 vol. Mouton, The Hague, 1973.
6. Jakobson, F.: Essais de linguistique générale, chap. 2, pp. 43–67. 1 vol. Ed. de minuit, Paris, 1963.

7. Jakobson, R.: Towards a linguistic typology of aphasic impairments. In: Disorders of language. 1 vol. Ciba Foundation Symposium, pp. 21–47. Churchill, London, 1964.

8. Lecours, A. R. & Lhermitte, F.: Phonemic paraphasias: linguistic structures and tentative hypotheses. Cortex /5/3: 193, 1969.

9. Lhermitte, F. Derouesne, J. & Signoret, J. L.: Analyse neuro-psychologique du syndrome frontal. Rev Neurol 127/4: 415, 1972.

10. Vignolo, L. A.: Evolution of aphasia and language rehabilitation: a retrospective exploratory study. Cortex 1: 344, 1964.

11. Luria, A. R.: Higher cortical functions in man. 1 vol. Harper and Row, New York, 1966.

12. Sabouraud, O., Gagnepain, J., & Sabouraud, A.: Vers une approche linguistique des problèmes de l'aphasie. I. Introduction. II. Essai d'une définition linguistique de l'aphasie de Broca. Rev de Neuro-Psych de l'Ouest 1 (2): 3, 1963.

13. Sabouraud, O., Gagnepain, J. & Chatel, M.: Qu'est-ce que l'Anarthie? Presse médicale, 79/15: 675, 1971.

14. Tissot, R., Mounin, G. & Lhermitte, F.: L'agrammatisme. 1 vol. Dessart, Bruxelles, 1973.

The language enriched, individual therapy program for aphasic patients

LEENA SALONEN

A multitude of programs and workbooks have been published for the purpose of improving the efficacy of rehabilitation of various aphasic disorders. It is, however, very difficult to design a coherent program which covers all aspects of language therapy in its many different forms and for different stages in the evolution of aphasia. Due to the complexity of the problem we must try to find such general linguistic, neuropsychological and pedagogical factors which integrate various procedures as logical parts of a whole.

In this paper the principles underlying a method called Language Enrichment Therapy (LET) are described. The therapeutic application of LET in its workbook (1, 2) is also explained.

Rationale

On the basis of experience gained by the use of the LET-method, contemporary views of the neurolinguistic characteristics of aphasia, their functional neuropsychological bases, (cf. 3, 4) the need for pedagogical approaches are interpreted in the following way:

1. Language behavior develops through a number of steps in which linguistic and cognitive functions interact gradually increasing in complexity. During development various linguistic levels—phonological, syntactic, semantic etc.—formed highly differentiated interacting systems which have parallel and hierarchical organizations and consist of sets of rules.

2. The activity of these systems is dependent on many systems of operations of other mental functions.

3. In aphasia, the unity and the integration of the interrelationships of linguistic and other functions are broken down and distorted.

4. Reacquisition of language in aphasia depends on reintegration of the linguistic systems and on restoration of the interactions between language and other mental functions. Rehabilitation should therefore:

— be aimed at restoring the interrelationships between language and other mental functions,

— build up the functions in the assumed order of their hierarchical organization,

— use preserved skills in the roles and relations they seem to have had at the various developmental and organizational stages of integration,
— apply learning theory principles, paying attention to the specific requirements of restorative pedagogics.

In aphasia, the interrelationships between language *systems* and their respective functional *operations* appear very clearly. In some cases the organization of a specific system seems to be well preserved, but because of a few lacking operations the patient cannot use the whole system. In other cases the organization of several systems is distorted, because a number of necessary operations are deficient. Perseveration, for example, is a typical operational distortion harmful for the functions of all language systems.

Language activities require numerous functional operations such as selection, comparison, sequencing, analysis, synthesis, retention, retrieval, etc. They produce nothing unless they are connected with a system and its content. For example, one cannot learn to recognize, to remember and to produce a single phoneme without a phonemic system of which it is a part. The phonemes, again, become meaningful only through their effect upon word meanings. Phonemes are also connected with other systems: the auditory-perceptive and the articulatory-motor.

Repetition, naming, and other similar functions which are traditionally tested in aphasia have no significance as *autonomous* activities. They are combinations of many other functional operations fulfilling some need of language development or usage. After becoming differentiated and automatic they serve, for their part, other functions as component operations. Only after gaining a high developmental level can they be used autonomously, detached from their original functional relations and roles. In restorative therapy such functions have to be linked to their original interrelations with other functions and reinforced in their role in the system.

The aphasic is not by himself able to analyze, control, or reconstruct partial functions and interactions. He adheres to preserved automatized activities but they become meaningless since they have lost connections to other ones. This is the case, for example, with "jargon" aphasia where the phonological system of expressive speech does not change, but the connections with the receptive phonological system and its operations have become diffuse.

The combination of component operations necessary for an activity like repetition requires a sequence of simultaneous and successive events. *Strategies* to perform such sequences are formed during the acquisition of language. Lacking operational skills make the former strategies useless.

Hierarchical organization appears to be a trait common to all mental functions, and the language functions seem, likewise, to develop and organize themselves hierarchically. For example, one unanimously accepted order of development is this: understanding precedes expressive speaking. A considerable number of expressions and words have to be interpreted and retained in some form before they can be built up to speech utterances. New information about some of the linguistic hierarchies—like that - of the syntactic system—has also been applied even to aphasia rehabilitation (5). Many functions seem to be organized from broad general classes into increasingly complex and differentiated ones, and learned effectively moving from approximate command of some general characteristics of the material to full mastery of its details.

The hierarchical structure of functional interactions breaks down in aphasia. Some high level functions may be preserved, some may be dissolved, inhibited or distorted, while still others appear to have regressed to a more primitive organizational level.

The LET-method is based on the conviction that the better we understand the hierarchical organization of the linguistic systems, the related mental functions and their interactions in learning, the more we can help the aphasic patient.

Pedagogical considerations of restorative therapy

On the basis of the working scheme discussed above some pedagogical principles need to be reformulated. If aphasic disorders are viewed as disintegration of interactions of linguistic and functional systems there are no logical grounds for drilling separate language skills without connecting them to other functions or without placing them in their due place among the other language activities.

Studies of childhood language development show that drilling a language skill is not successful until the child has reached the required cognitive maturation. The aphasic, likewise, can reacquire the mastery of a specific skill, only when required other functions have reached the necessary level of integration.

Word production exercises do not seem sensible before the patient has a relatively clear idea of the meaning of these words. Neither does auditory training as such yield positive results unless it is planned with regard to a step-by-step reorganization of language systems. The same applies to attempts to restore any particular purpose of language usage, e.g. language needed in the hospital or in the bank, etc.

In general, good results can not be expected by exercising any one single language function which is not integrated into the functional systems of language. However, when introduced through proper phases of relations, a whole functional scheme seems to be restored and generalized to various fields of use independent of the material rehearsed.

A diffuse and distorted system cannot assume its role in the organization. In such a case the operations to be restored do not have the necessary bases of integration. The reorganization of linguistic systems and the restoration of functional operations are the two main lines along which language therapy should proceed either simultaneously or in alternating turns.

In this method an activated, organized system of understanding word meanings is regarded as the foundation to which all other systems and operations are anchored. Therefore, the first stage of therapy involves systematic *activation* of this system using a rich variety of exercises of comprehension.

Unfortunately, our knowledge of the processes of language reception in aphasia is deficient. It seems that certainly problems of selection, perseveration, dissociation of word meanings, and impaired retention are operational factors which reduce the efficiency of the decoding of language. The understanding of spoken language in aphasia appears to proceed stage by stage from very general undifferentiated ideas about the content of short redundant sentences to the precise understanding of the meanings of the details. This development is likely to be dependent on the re-occurrence of the expressions and their parts in changing contexts of meaning and structure. Exact and sustained understanding of single words is a rather advanced stage of reception, and a very important prerequisite for the detailed understanding of complex sentences.

The development of receptive abilities can be assumed to involve a close linkage with the development of other mental functions which are also needed for the planning of expressive speech. Therefore, most aphasics seem to need exercises of comprehension. Even the patients who appear to comprehend speech relatively well benefit from such exercises due to the new *orientation* towards understanding they gain. This means that the former automatized processes of understanding are transferred gradually to a more *conscious* activity, which enables the patient to analyze language for expressive purposes.

Only firmly established operations can be integrated into an *operational system*. For this reason it is beneficial to train each operation for a sufficiently long time in the same form using it always in new contexts. This procedure enables rules to develop. For example, in picture-choice exercises of comprehension the syntactic structure of the sentence remains the same long enough while the component words are continuously changed, and the patient gradually forms several rules involving e.g. sentence structure, possible meaningful combinations of words, and forms of associative relations of the items to the pictures.

The operations of all fields of language functions need to be gradually strengthened in the same way so that performance becomes a firm and flexible routine. Operations are built up on other operations, their elements are changed, they are used in different contexts and roles, and they can be integrated as a component into a new skill. The efficacy of even the most elementary operations is important as recovery progresses. Therefore the same operations are taken up periodically for renewed training in order to raise functions up to the level permitted by the development of other supportive operations.

The LET-method

The LET-method is implemented in a workbook based on the principles described above. These guidelines and detailed instructions are presented in an understandable format for nonprofessionals, and the structure was planned to be as convenient as possible. All required therapy material is included.

The LET-material includes also *a screening-test* with which the clinician can assess the central areas of language functions. The test consists of main exercises from the LET-material and thus provides a direct connection between test results and therapy.

The workbook

The workbook consists of three parts: 1) a set of pictures illustrating 160 basic words, 2) a set of language units, and 3) exercise instructions.

The pictures are presented on pages in groups of eight. Room is left for the corresponding examples from the language units, written on paper strips, to be inserted between them, as seen in Fig. 1.

In the 28 language units, the basic words are continually utilized in new connections and contexts. This takes place in groups of words, in sentences, and stories, and in different subject and usage connections. The vocabulary is thus cumulatively enriched to include 6,000 words. The units consist of selected patterns of language structures, usages and functional properties. By transforming, modifying, combining, and expanding them, an endless variety of structures can be produced to serve various purposes, and yet they always have some kind of connection to the basic words.

The instructions offer a great number of commonly used methods, as well as procedures described by A. R. Luria (3, 6, 7). The estimated order in which the operations required for different skills should be trained is indicated, and the relations to other operations, and possibilities of transformation are pointed out.

Basic techniques

Comprehension. All examples of the 28 language units corresponding to the 160 basic words can be used as picture-choice tasks, as seen in Fig. 2. Each of the basic words is thus combined with other words, structures, associations, semantic relations, etc. in a considerable number of ways even in receptive exercises. Therapy is always started with the activation of receptive skills using a few of the main units, but even later on, before training of other functions, the corresponding unit is first given as a comprehension task using picture-choice. To be sure that the meaning content of the items used for the training of expression is understood, this training is also always done in connection with the pictures.

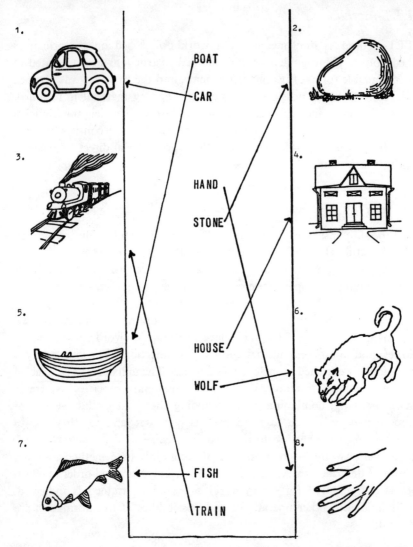

Fig. 1. The LET-method uses a set of illustrations of 160 basic words which linked in numerous ways with a variety of linguistic context, and combinations cumulate up to a vocabulary of 6,000 words.

Expression. The same language items are used as stimuli for expression. They can be intoned, repeated or combined in the beginning of the therapy. Later on they are gradually transformed, modified, and expanded for various purposes. The basic goal kept in mind in all phases of therapy is to support the patient's intentional speaking.

Reading and writing. The LET-material is used as visual picture-choice exercises for reading, and all exercises of expression are produced in written form for writing.

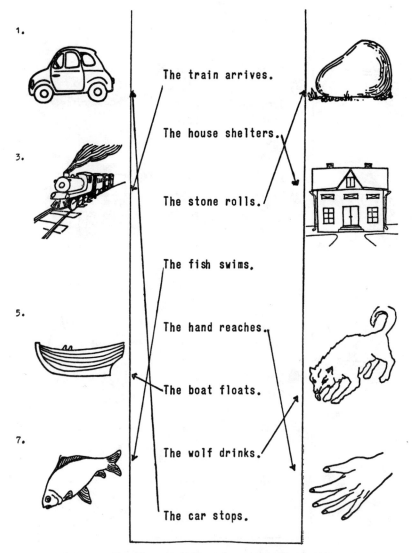

Fig. 2. Receptive abilities are rehabilitated using picture-choice of a great variety of linguistic items. The subprograms for receptive training are organized to proceed in a hierarchical manner which depends on the patients' individual style of learning.

Activation of the language systems. The reorganization of the system of word-meaning relationships takes place varying comprehension exercises systematically. Later on other systems are organized on the basis of this basic system.

Functional operations. All operations at any level are made firm by using the same operation at one time in connection with all 160 language items, as seen in Fig. 3.

Hierarchical order of progression. Varying systematically the structures of

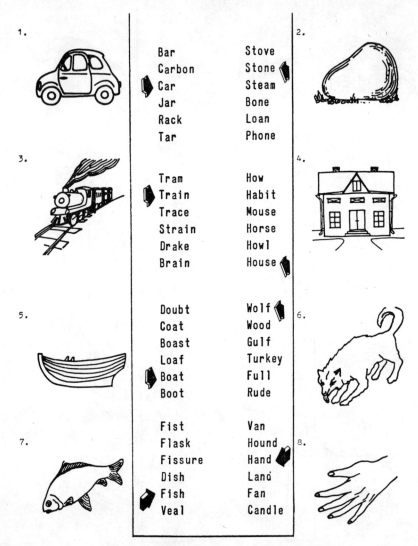

Fig. 3. The manner of using the given language items can be varied in a controlled way in search for helpful procedures. For example, in conduction aphasia, the increase in the accuracy of detecting right and wrong auditory stimuli from a group of words which sound alike was found to effectively restore the repetition of the intended words.

operations the patient's individual order of learning is searched for and controlled by clear evidence of an increase in correct performances in each modification of the subprograms, as seen in Fig. 4.

Intersystemic interactions. The intersystemic interactions are primarily supported by the use of the same language items in the rehabilitation of various functions. For example, items comprehended in detail are a good source for exercises of memory.

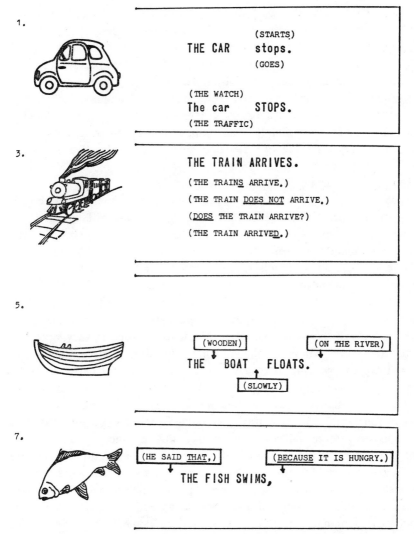

1.

(STARTS)
THE CAR stops.
(GOES)

(THE WATCH)
The car STOPS.
(THE TRAFFIC)

3.

THE TRAIN ARRIVES.
(THE TRAINS ARRIVE.)
(THE TRAIN DOES NOT ARRIVE.)
(DOES THE TRAIN ARRIVE?)
(THE TRAIN ARRIVED.)

5.

(WOODEN)   (ON THE RIVER)
THE BOAT FLOATS.
(SLOWLY)

7.

(HE SAID THAT,)   (BECAUSE IT IS HUNGRY.)
THE FISH SWIMS,

Fig. 4. The language items can be transformed in numerous ways, but each transformation is performed in connection with all the 160 basic words in order to stabilize the necessary functional operations and linguistic rules.

Experiences and observations

The LET-method is still in the process of deveopment. Up till now the primary interest has, therefore, been to find out some principles upon which a coherent therapy could be planned. Only some tentative observations made during a few years of clinical application of the method can be described here. Later on, these hypotheses, will require more careful study.

1. The use of a comprehensive and controlled aphasia rehabilitation program seems to yield new insights into the specific language learning characteristics of aphasia. In addition to its original purpose—to give the

therapists a rich variety of ready-to-use language exercises—it can be used for clinical experimentation, particularly for longitudinal studies.

2. Each form of aphasia requires, of course, concentration on the training of specific language areas. Still it appears that some basic steps necessary for the reacquisition of language are shared by most aphasics. These steps seem to reflect general hierarchical levels of the organization of linguistic processing. They cannot be overlooked: a steady progress in recovery depends on the gradual growth of mastery of these steps in their due order. However, the methods necessary for reaching these subgoals vary according to the form of aphasia and a patient's individual manner of learning.

3. Language relearning in aphasia seems to be based on the restoration of various operational skills and on the reorganization of linguistic and cognitive systems and their interactions. Therefore, the selection of language items in a program is not as such learned and used by the patients. On the contrary, the language material in a program is an indispensable instrument for the reorganization of linguistic processing rather than merely something to be learned or memorized.

This observation is based on the comparison between the listed vocabulary of the LET and the expressive speech of patients treated using the LET-material. Although the same basic linguistic items are used in varying forms, contexts, and modifications in all modalities, this does not seem to restrict the growth of the patients' language repertoire. The author believes, on the contrary, that this approach has the advantage of reinforcing in a concentrated and systematic way the functional bases of linguistic processing.

4. The functional and operational characteristics of linguistic processing seem to deserve more attention, both in evaluating the outcome of the treatment and in constructing rehabilitation programs. A collection of language rehabilitation material for aphasics should represent a sufficiently wide variety of linguistic items which can be combined and modified in a systematic way for various linguistic, communicative and therapeutic purposes. However, the operational manner in which these meaning contexts are treated is of primary importance.

5. The stimuli employed in language therapy should be chosen in a way which not only elicits correct responses but also aids the development of efficacy, speed, accuracy, and applicability of the restored operations. Pure drill is not efficient unless the patient possesses the necessary skills for integrating the drilled material into his operational system. Drilling is, however, often needed to increase the functional efficacy of the operations restored by other techniques.

6. Language reacquisition in aphasia involves continuous qualitative changes in the interaction between linguistic and cognitive systems, their operational bases, and of the necessary strategies. In aphasia rehabilitation, at all its stages, it is therefore a continual challenge to observe the changing conditions and possibilities and readjust the therapeutic approach accordingly.

References

1. Salonen, L.: Regain your speaking ability: a rehabilitation guide for aphasic patients (in Finnish). Koulun Erityispalvelu, Helsinki, 1977.
2. Salonen, L.: A new set of language retraining materials for aphasic patients. International Association of Logopedics and Phoniatrics Congress Proceedings, Copenhagen 1977, pp. 501–509. Special-Paedagogisk Forlag, Herning, 1978.
3. Luria, A. R.: Traumatic Aphasia. Mouton, The Hague, 1970.
4. Luria, A. R.: Aphasia reconsidered. Cortex 8: 34, 1972.
5. Crystal, D., Fletcher, P. & Garman, M.: The Grammatical Analysis of Language Disability. A Procedure for Assessment and Remediation. Arnold, London, 1976.
6. Luria, A. R.: Restoration of Function after Brain Injury. Pergamon Press, London, 1964.
7. Luria, A. R., Naydin, V. L., Tsvetkova, L. S. & Vinarskaya, E. N.: Restoration of higher cortical function following local brain damage. In: P. J. Vinken & W. G. Bruyn (eds.), Handbook of Neurology, vol. 3, pp. 368–433. North Holland Publ Co, Amsterdam, 1969.

Education of speech therapists, especially in aphasia: Experiences from Sweden

GUNNAR BJUGGREN AND EVA IHRE

Phoniatrics became a medical speciality in the nineteen thirties. Speech therapy was developed through personal contributions here and there in the country, among other places in Gothenburg which is now the seat of our symposium. However, this development was greatly delayed, since the training of professionals in the field was neglected. Not until the sixties were our two separate lines of training constituted. One is the special line of Speech Therapy at the Teachers' College (lärarhögskolan) for 1-year additional training in logopedics for teachers, intending to become speech therapists in the school. The other line comprises a 3-year academic program for the training of Logopedists. The latter program started in Stockholm in 1964 with a productive capacity of 10 logopedists per year. In the beginning a shortage of competent teachers and other difficulties set a narrow limit on productivity.

Heavy demands for a more frequent production led to an analysis of requirements in 1967 (Hans Lindholm) and, in consequence, to the training of further 10 logopedists at the University of Lund. In the 1968 Educational Commission (U 68) the productivity required was estimated to about 50 logopedists per year. After a two step evaluation (Gunnar Bjuggren) in 1974 and 1977 (the latter stage in collaboration with the National Board of Health and Welfare on "The need of Logopedists in the public medical service") was carried out, the total admission to the training has already been increased to an average of 32 students per year and the National Board of Universities and Colleges has suggested a gradual rise to 48 students per year.

Gothenburg is close to becoming the next in turn to start a training course. Assuming that the whole country has need of logopedists on the same level as the region of medical care, which is best provided for, the evaluations mentioned were based on the logopedist-resources found in this region at the time of investigation, as well as on the future needs of the same region, estimated for both short and long term needs. With the present proposed capacity of admission the number of logopedists in the 80's will increase from 3 to 8 logopedists/100,000 inhabitants and in the 90's to 12 logopedists/100,000 inhabitants, which is on a par with the present capacity of the U.S.

The nervous system carries important functions, with respect to communication through spoken language. Lesions and affections of a neurological nature thus often lead to speech and language disorders. Different kinds of treatment of these neurological cases have to be an integrated whole with phoniatric and logopedic care as a part. Among these cases, aphasics make up a large group.

In accordance with the definition, an aphasic is a person suffering from aphasia. However, in the clinical reality the conditions are more complex than that, since besides aphasia there are generally one or several of a variety of symptoms, which need to be handled through a team approach. Therefore, it seems more accurate to talk about the treatment and rehabilitation of aphasics than aphasia rehabilitation.

In the very beginning it became evident to the leader of the course (Bjuggren), that the framework of the three year training program for logopedists was too narrow. It was also unsatisfactory that one was compelled to accept courses in phonetics and psychology (pedagogies), which were conceived for other educational lines. This disadvantage, however, didn't manifest itself very much as long as these subjects were taken before the admission bar, since many of the applicants because of competition had redundant qualifications. However, the different courses of the 3-year program became an administrative unity and redundant studies in these subjects no longer were useful for applicants. It was evident that the 1-semester psychology course was insufficient. This fall semester, a qualitative improvement will at last take place with a basic psychology course specially adapted to the training of logopedics. It comprises General Psychology (5 points), Methodology (6 points), Personality Psychology (6 points), Social Psychology (3 points). This course will, among other things, give basic knowledge in the most common methods of evaluation and research within the psychology field.

During the last three semesters, which is devoted to Logopedics (60 points) the students are prepared for the task of treating neurological cases. This course includes among other things: Anatomy and physiology (3 points), which aims at giving "a deeper knowledge of the central nervous system as well as certain parts of the peripheral system" and at which "special attention is given to neurophysiological testing methods and the information these methods give about the function of the speech apparatus"; Neurology and neurological rehabilitation (18 lecture hours); Cerebral palsy (10 hours), Psychiatry and Psychotherapy (30 hours); Childpsychiatry (16 hours), Social Medicine (6 hours).

Centrally conditioned language disorders (8 points) does not apply only to adults but also children with cerebral palsy. Under this headline you also find "Therapy oriented evaluation and testing methods", "Aphasia and dysarthia therapy, its prerequisites, principles and execution." Furthermore, "Verbal A D L training" and "The connection of therapy to *social measures* to introduce treated aphasics into an atmosphere of contact and communication".

Clinical work under supervision takes up 12 weeks. This takes place, in part, at the Department of Phoniatrics at Huddinge University Hospital, where the students practice treating aphasics individually as well as in groups. During the last six weeks different kinds of dysarthric patients are treated. During the periods of clinical practice the students are divided into groups of two.

At the Dept of Phoniatrics during the whole period the students take part in the treatment of out-patients for 2 days/week and $2\frac{1}{2}$ hours/day, out of which $1\frac{1}{2}$ hours are devoted to therapy and the remaining 1 hour to supervised casework, professional reports, testing procedures, relevant literature, how to inform the patient and his family and how the logopedist collaborates in the rehabilitation team. Furthermore the students describe the purpose of therapy and give suggestions for treatment programs. For further 3 hours/week they practice in rehabilitation groups.

A neurologist is available for consultation upon request by the supervisor.

At the rehabilitation centers the students work closely with occupational therapists, physical therapists and social workers.

Seminars are part of the theoretical education. At the seminars journal articles on neurological language and speech disorders are reported by the students.

Students are examined at the end of the 12 weeks neurology section of the course of logopedics on the assigned literature and clinical principles.

In a memorandum to the National Board of Universities and Colleges a Phoniatric-Neurologic Committee at the Sahlgrenska Hospital in Gothenburg presented "Qualitative aspects on Aphasia rehabilitation and the training of logopedists". The opinion stated is that the training of logopedists in all essential phases of aphasia rehabilitation gives the fundamental knowledge but that this knowledge—with the exception of linguistics and proficiency in dysarthria therapy—is in need of deepening.

One of us (Bjuggren) is to a great extent responsible for the design of the training program for logopedists and the other (Ihre) is as a teacher involved in its current execution at Huddinge Hospital. In this lecture we have attempted to give a description of the training program and particularly of the way it is executed when it comes to neurological language and speech disorders.

Indeed, although the description is brief we hope that we have shown that the neurology section of the course of logopedics is an ambitious organization and holds a prominent position in the program. At the same time we have pointed out that the 3-year frame is too limited. At an early stage it became evident that it would need to be supplemented by additional training, which was expressed in the standard syllabus, valid from 1972 on: "The course of Logopedics can within the given time limit give only fundamental knowledge of the methods applied within respective areas of medical care and social welfare". In principle we agree with the committee but maybe not completely concerning its evaluation of separate parts of the present training. However, this complex problem can be clarified within the near future, when hopefully the training of logopedists will also start in Gothenburg and the committee will thus have access to local study material.

Education of aphasia therapists in Norway—facts and future plans

KRISTIAN KRISTIANSEN AND IVAR REINVANG

The treatment of aphasia is intimately related to the rehabilitation of the stroke patient and of the brain injured individual in general. It can thus hardly be regarded as a separate clinical discipline but must be integrated in a retraining program. On the other hand—as a neurologist or a neurosurgeon, as a nurse or a physiotherapist—one has to admit a painful inability in dealing with the different aspects of aphasia. Even a well trained psychologist will as a rule refrain from the complex task of understanding and treating an aphasic patient.

Before the second world war there was very little interest in Norway, or in the rest of the world, in the therapeutic aspects of aphasic disorders. Systems of classification were elaborated also in our country. Monrad-Krohn's well organized scheme of examination was repeatedly published in his widely distributed textbook "Clinical Examination of the Nervous System". Norwegian neurologists of the older generation remember the many hours spent with filling in the questionnaire which was required in every case of aphasic disturbance. Monrad-Krohn was also interested in the altered prosody of language or speech melody in patients with aphasia (2). This interest was initiated during the German occupation of Norway after the admission to the Neurological Department of a female patient, who in spite of a partial aphasia, was able to explain her situation. A couple of weeks before she had been hit in the left side of her head by a bomb fragment during an air raid on Oslo. She complained of the difficulty in finding the right words, but particularly of being regarded by her fellow Norwegians as a German because of a peculiar change of her accent. Another Norwegian neurologist, Hjalmar Torp, was interested in the linguistic aspects of aphasia, perhaps due to an influence from his father, Professor Alf Torp, a prominent linguist at the University of Oslo.

During the past 20–30 years the treatment and rehabilitation of hemiplegic patients with aphasia have been the joint efforts of nurses, physiotherapists, occupational therapists and speech therapists—in Norway named logopedists. In the hospitals the medical supervision has been carried out by neurologists if a neurological department has been established, otherwise by internists, or—in a few hospitals—by specialists in geriatrics and social medicine. The specialty of physical medicine and rehabilitation has been poorly developed and there is no chair in this field in our four medical schools.

The schools for physiotherapy, occupational therapy and nursing give only a brief orientation on aphasia for their students, not exceeding a few hours teaching. The speech therapists have a basic training as primary school teachers with an additional 2 years course at the Postgraduate Teacher Training Center of Special Education. For those students who choose aphasia as a particular subject, a theoretical course of 40 hours and two weeks of practice at an institution with aphasic patients are required. A third year of study has recently been added for the students at this institution. This year shall be devoted mainly to writing a thesis on a topic relevant to the student's chief field of interest.

In our medical schools there is no organized teaching in aphasia. The first postgraduate course in aphasia for neurologists and neurosurgeons was held in September 1978. Basic courses in psychology at our universities do not include material on aphasia.

In 1963 the Norwegian Council on Heart and Vascular Diseases, a section of the National Health Association, selected cerebro-vascular diseases as the main theme for their annual publicity week. Since then there has been a growing interest in Norway for the rehabilitation of stroke patients. The never failing interest of Dr T. Gedde-Dahl, the secretary-general of the National Health Association, has been most important for the progress of the plans. In 1969 a joint conference including linguists, psychologists, speech therapists and medical doctors, was organized in Oslo with the purpose of stimulating the inter-disciplinary cooperation for the study and teaching of aphasia (1). Four years later, in 1973, an institute for aphasia and stroke was established through financial support from the National Health Association, at Sunnaas Hospital, a 250 bed rehabilitation center, situated just outside Oslo and closely related to Ullevål Hospital, which is one of the teaching hospitals of the University of Oslo. As head of the institute was appointed one of the authors (I. R.), who has a basic education in psychology from the University of Oslo and two years as a post-graduate fellow at the Massachusetts Institute of Technology with Professor H. L. Teuber. From January 1977 the intitute has been recognized by the state authorities as a section of the hospital, which means that it is incorporated in the hospital budget.

In Sunnaas Hospital about 50 patients with aphasia are seen each year, thus providing the Institute with a sufficient study and teaching material. Published studies based on this material are those by Reinvang (4, 5, 6), Reinvang and Graves (7) and Reinvang et al. (8).

Besides research activities the main task during the first few years has been to give courses on language pathology and principles of treatment. In the fall of 1974 the first 3 months' course in aphasia was organized for nurses, physiotherapists, occupational therapists and speech therapists. Members of these professions were considered well qualified for further training in aphasia. It is our hope that those who have completed the courses, will serve as distributors of knowledge at their places of work in different parts of the country.

Future plans

The beneficial effects of specific speech therapy in aphasic patients have been demonstrated by several aphasiologists. The plans for development in this field in Norway must consider the fact that the majority of such patients are widely scattered across the thinly populated country, that only a small number will be treated—and only for short periods—in the regional hospitals attached to the universities, and that the long-term therapy will have to be carried out in nursing homes, in homes for the aged, or in the patients' own homes. The primary aim must be to give barely sufficient competence to interested persons recruited from health personnel groups. To this end the duration of the courses at the aphasia institute has been reduced to about three weeks. Short courses are more attractive for the students and also more easily financed by the local authorities responsible for health care in the counties and the municipal districts. Personnel trained in such brief courses would be assumed to qualify for carrying out therapeutic tasks under supervision, and for screening cases which should be referred to more highly trained personnel for closer evaluation. Through publicity campaigns in daily newspapers, radio and television, attention should be focused on the possibilities of rehabilitation for patients with aphasia.

The next step is to establish a central registry for aphasic patients in order to obtain necessary data on the need of retraining. Based on Petlund's study (3) from 1970 on prevalence and invalidity from stroke in one of the counties, the number of disabled stroke patients in Norway is roughly estimated at 7,500. The number among those suffering from aphasia amenable to therapy is unknown, as is also the number of patients with aphasia after head injuries and other brain diseases.[1]

Another equally important task for the Institute of Aphasia and Stroke is to organize cooperation between representatives of the professions that may potentially influence the development of aphasia research in Norway. An association corresponding to the Academy of Aphasia in the United States is desirable in every language group. Perhaps the close relation and the similarities between the Danish, Norwegian and Swedish tongues may allow the creation of a Scandinavian joint enterprise in this field. An agreement on terminology, on methods of examination, on basic patterns for treatment and criteria for selection of patients amenable to a therapeutic approach, is one of the first important subjects for discussion in such an organization. A more limited inter-disciplinary group should be appointed to prepare a report and recommendations which could form the basis for discussions in a larger forum.[2]

---

[1] In December 1977 a laboratory for aphasia was inaugurated at the County Hospital of Lillehammer.
[2] This proposal was discussed during the seminar. A group of representatives from the Scandinavian countries was elected, and is expected to deliver a report in 1980.

The effects of new methods of treatment will have to be tested on suitable patients. To increase the capacity for aphasia research along these lines it is imperative to establish institutes for aphasia and stroke research. Teams comprising neurologists, neuropsychologists, neurolinguists and aphasia therapists must be appointed full time employees of such institutions to secure continuity and to keep abreast of new techniques of investigation and therapy.

References

1. Hartviksen, K., Gulbrandsen, G. B., Reinvang, I. & Vogt, H.: Afasi. Forskning og behandlingsmuligheter. Tidsskr Nor Laegeforen 89: 1713, 1969.
2. Monrad-Krohn, G. H.: Dysprosody or altered melody of language. Brain 70: 405, 1947.
3. Petlund, C. F.: Prevalence and Invalidity from Stroke in Aust-Agder County of Norway. Universitetsforlaget, Oslo, 1970.
4. Reinvang, I.: Aleksi uten agrafi. Tidsskr Nor Laegeforen 95: 1971, 1975.
5. Reinvang, I.: Task variables affecting short term memory in aphasics. Paper presented at the meeting of the International Neuropsychology Society, Oxford, 1977 a.
6. Reinvang, I.: Language recovery in aphasia. Developments 3 to 6 months after stroke. Paper presented at present symposium, 1977 b.
7. Reinvang, I. & Graves, R.: A basic aphasia examination. Scand J Rehab Med 7: 129, 1975.
8. Reinvang, I., Hjeltnes, N. & Guvaag, S. P.: Afasibehandling av hjerneslagpasienter. Tidsskr Nor Laegeforen 96: 1421, 1976.

The pattern of cortical activation during speech and listening in normals and different types of aphasic patients as revealed by regional cerebral blood flow (rCBF)

ERIK SKINHØJ AND BO LARSEN

Sherrington's old concept: Coupling between neuronal activity, cerebral metabolism and cerebral blood flow is now established within certain controllable conditions (2). Thus measurement of regional cerebral blood flow (rCBF) yields a new tool for the study of human brain activity in the normal as well as in the diseased brain. With the until now most advanced equipment for rCBF measurement designed by Niels A. Lassen and co-workers: The computerized dynamic gamma camera it is possible simultaneously to determine rCBF in 254 cortical areas using the intracarotid [133]Xenon injection method. Concerning the mathematical and physical principles of this method, the technical details of the equipment, sensitivity, power of resolution and stereotactic localization I must refer to our original papers (1, 3), but in a way all this is illustrated in Fig. 1 showing the activation by a discrimination test made by foot, hand and mouth respectively.

The resting pattern of brain activity is very constant with a frontal hyperemia as shown in Fig. 2, there is no difference between the dominant and the nondominant hemisphere. This in spite of the fact that the absolute flow values in normals at rest have a very wide range: 36–80 ml/100 g/min, simply reflecting the concept of a "resting brain" is an abstraction. As long as you live the human brain is never resting.

Listening

During listening, in the present series listening to onomatopoeia such as splash, bow-wow, buzz etc., i.e. the simplest form of afferent language the resting flow pattern is significantly changed in both hemispheres as shown in Fig. 3. The pictures are superimposed from 10 normal subjects but the pattern in all of them was the same: Increased activity in the posterior part of the superior temporal lobe—corresponding to the primary auditory cortex—to a certain degree spreading to the surrounding association area in the parietal and the occipital lobe, corresponding rather well to the old Wernicke centre. Beside that an activation is seen in the frontal lobe. Listening with the left or the right ear did not change the pattern neither in the dominant nor in the non-dominant hemisphere.

Automatic speech

Fig. 4 shows a pattern of activation during automatic speech such as naming the months or the days of the week. The most striking activation is now seen in the primary motor-sensory area for muscles involved in speech but beside that from the supplementary motor area and in the Wernicke centre as well. Listening to your own voice is a needed feedback for speech. Furthermore, an activation is seen in the frontal lobe but with a different localization as the one seen during listening. This pattern of activation during speech is in accordance with a cortical speech map of Penfield and co-workers based on electrical stimulation during brain operation in local anaesthesia (Fig. 5). The most astonishing in our studies is that the non-dominant hemisphere in normal man takes an equal part in language as does the dominant, maybe a little more diffuse and widespread.

Studies during aphasia

Beside our normal studies we examined a series of aphasic patients realizing of course that we to some extent exceed the basic limitations of our methods, f. ex. the fact that the partition coefficient between Xe in blood and normal brain tissue components—entering our mathematical model—is no longer quantitatively valid in cases of tumors, infarcts etc. In spite of this the results seem to give some interesting information. I cannot go into details but only show the summarizing Fig. 6 demonstrating that in all cases of fluent aphasia a dysfunction is seen corresponding to the Wernicke centre and in all cases of non fluent or motor aphasia the primary motor centres of speech are impaired. In cases of global aphasia the dysfunction is very widespread. It may be added that in some of the cases other examinations such as CT-scan, angiography, EEG etc. did not reveal focal abnormalities. In other cases the anatomical abnormalities were much less than the functional disturbances as

---

Fig. 1. Flow pattern during discrimination test with mouth, hand and foot respectively.

Fig. 2. The normal hemispheric pattern of flow distribution at rest, average of 12 subjects studied in the left hemisphere (upper) and 15 subjects studied in the right hemisphere (lower).

Fig. 3. The average changes of the hemispheric pattern of flow distribution from rest to listening in 9 left hemispheres and 9 right hemispheres.

Fig. 4. The average changes of the hemispheric pattern of flow distribution from rest to automatic speech in 8 left hemispheres and 8 right hemispheres.

Fig. 5. Summary of areas in which stimulation may interfere with speech or produce vocalization in the dominant hemisphere (Penfield and Rasmussen 1949).

Fig. 6. Cortical areas with impaired rCBF in different types of aphasia.

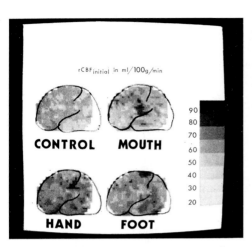

rCBF$_{initial}$ in ml/100g/min

CONTROL MOUTH

HAND FOOT

90
80
70
60
50
40
30
20

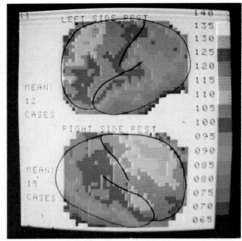

2

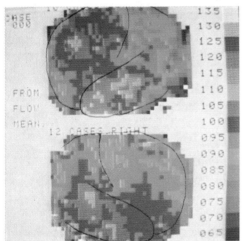

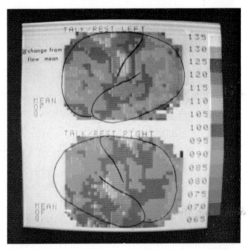

4

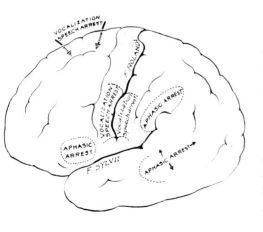

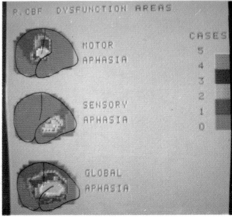

6

revealed by the rCBF studies. This involves the basic fact that rCBF measurements are functional and not anatomical studies and that the sensitivity of this method is much higher than in the conventional methods for the study of brain activity.

It is worth mentioning that in case of aphasia—or other focal cortical lesions —an attempt to overcome the disability often results in an activation in cortical areas ordinarily not involved in these functions. This may explain the fatigue often clinically observed during training of the aphasic patient.

It must be admitted that it is difficult at the present time to see the direct therapeutic use of our studies but nevertheless all rational therapy must be based upon expanding biological and physiological knowledge and we hope that our studies represent a little step in that direction.

References

1. Olesen, J., Paulson, O. B. & Lassen, N. A.: Regional cerebral blood flow in man determined by the initial slope of the clearance of intra-artrially injected [133]Xe. Stroke 2: 519, 1971.
2. Raichle, M. E., Grubb, R. L., Mokhtar, H. G., Eechling, J. O. & Ter-Pogossian, M. M.: Correlation between regional cerebral blood flow and oxydative metabolism. Arch Neurol 33: 523, 1976.
3. Sveinsdottir, E., Larsen, B., Rommer, P. & Lassen, N. A.: A multidector scintillation camera with 254 channels. J Nucl Med 18: 168, 1977.

Notes on the anatomical basis
of pure alexia and of color anomia[1]

ANTONIO R. DAMASIO

A list of current questions regarding the anatomical basis of alexia and of color anomia, would read as follows: What is the significance of a lesion in the splenium of the corpus callosum in the production of alexia and of color anomia? Assuming that the splenium does have a role, what portion of it, dorsal or ventral, is related to the production of alexia or of color anomia, or of both? What areas of the left occipital lobe, when damaged, seem crucial for alexia and color anomia to appear? And: Is the ventral outflow of the occipital lobe different from the dorsal? Which of the two, when damaged, produces alexia, color anomia or both?

The question regarding the role of the splenium is the older one and the problem is often misrepresented in modern writings on the subject. Déjerine is generally quoted as calling attention to the role of the lesion in the splenium when he did exactly the opposite in his seminal paper of 1892. Although his patient did have a lesion in the splenium in addition to a lesion of the mesial cortex of the occipital lobe and of its underlying white matter, Déjerine actually argued that the whole syndrome could be parsimoniously explained by the occipital lesion with little need to invoke the splenium. ["La lésion des masses blanches sous-jacentes au lobe occipital gauche était assez étendue, puisqu'elle atteignait l'épendyme ventriculaire, pour que nous puissions admettre que les fibres qui relient le pli courbe gauche aux deux lobes occipitaux aient été intéressées, et sans que nous avons besoin de faire intervenir une seconde lésion, la petite lésion siégeant dans le bourrelet du corps calleux."] The case of Brissaud in 1900 had similar pathologic findings and again no emphasis was given to the splenium. What both Déjerine and Brissaud did was to insist on disconnection (between primary visual areas and a "visuo-verbal" center in the angular gyrus) as the mechanism capable of explaining the syndrome, regardless of where exactly disconnection would take place. It was Foix and Hillemand, in 1925, who called attention to the possible role of the lesion in the corpus callosum proper by demonstrating a patient *without* alexia in whom the pathological findings were similar to the ones reported by Déjerine in his famous case but *without* splenial involvement. The authors argued convincingly that the lack of splenial lesion was responsible for the

[1] Part of a paper read at the 1977 Meeting of the Research Group of Aphasia of the World Federation of Neurology, Göteborg, Sweden.

patient's preserved reading ability while the addition of such a lesion would have produced a reading defect.

By and large the remarkable observations and conclusions of these French neurologists have stood the test of time and have been replicated in nearly all of the well documented cases of alexia, color anomia or both (for the standard description and post mortem correlation of the combined syndrome, see Geschwind and Fusillo, 1966). Nevertheless, there are exceptional cases and a few patients have been shown to have pure alexia in the absence of a lesion in the splenium. How can one account for such instances? First of all it is important to consider what the report of lack of lesions in the splenium can mean. Often it simply betrays ambiguous use of terminology. If the concept of splenium is restricted to denote the midline region of the caudal portion of the corpus callosum, a lesion in the prolongation of the callosum into the hemisphere at the level of the *forceps major* will be considered an occipital lobe lesion and not a lesion of the splenium. That is obviously erroneous, since the functional significance of a lesion of the callosal outflow, at that particular level, is probably similar to that of a lesion in the callosal midline, at least as far as the reading process is concerned (the same might not be true for other processes, such as color naming, for instance). In other words if the correct anatomical concept is used, few patients with pure alexia fail to show a splenial lesion though not all of them need have it close to the midline. It is noteworthy that in the original case of Déjerine there was both a small lesion in the ventral portion of the splenium and a larger lesion in the depth of the hemisphere which severed interhemispheric connections in addition to occipito-parietal projections. Finally, it appears that in some cases, the splenium, even if correctly considered to mean "midline" and "outflow", may be partially spared. What sort of lesion has been found to associate with alexia in those cases? The common denominator appears to be the partial or complete damage of the outflow from some regions of the left occipital cortex, particularly those in the peristriate belt, in which interhemispheric pathways articulate. Greenblatt has argued this point in a recent paper (1976) on the basis of a case of alexia in which the callosum was possibly intact. His contentions are based on angiographic and neurosurgical data but supported by previous demonstration of the importance of subcortical occipital structures in a post-mortem study (1973). In that case of pure alexia the patient had neither hemianopia nor color anomia, and the cortex of the occipital lobe was spared although the lingual and fusiform gyri were undercut by a lesion of the white matter. The dorsal outflow of the occipital cortex was intact. The splenium was involved in its inferior aspect. Thus, it is possible that damage to certain visual information pathways such as the ones mentioned by Greenblatt occurring after left and right visual inputs have been integrated and processed (e.g. in structures of the lingual and fusiform gyri), correlates with pure alexia. Furthermore, the ventral component of such pathways might be more consistently associated with alexia.

The picture which emerges from the different placing and combination of lesions associated with alexia, underscores the complexity of the visual processing system on which reading depends. We are not dealing with the interruption of one single important pathway bringing visual information to one reading operator, but rather with the disruption of the stepwise analysis and modification of certain features of visual information along a chain of neural processors which will eventually produce reading. Most probably more than one hierarchy of occipital cortical processors is involved, appropriately interconnected, receiving visual information from both visual fields. A predominant outflow, possibly ventral occipital, then articulates in structures of the inferior parietal region and upper posterior temporal lobe.

It is interesting to reflect now on the anatomical data related to color anomia. Since the publication of Geschwind and Fusillo's case (1966) several observations came to light which implement the disconnection model proposed by Geschwind. Cummings, Hurvitz and Perl (1970) reported a patient with pure alexia in whom the classical anatomical features (left occipital lesion plus lesion in the splenium) were present but color naming was normal. Detailed observation of the splenium revealed that only its ventral portion had been damaged (that is often the case since part of this structure is a watershed zone and the dorsum can quite commonly be spared) and the authors, and other researchers since then, have suggested that the preservation of some fibers could have been enough to allow right hemisphere visual input to reach parietal structures and thus permit color naming. Recently Ajax and coworkers (1977) have contended that the more dorsal elements of the splenium subserve color naming while only the ventral third is vital for the reading process. Although that is possible, we would like to point out at least one alternative mechanism to explain the preservation of color naming: Color naming may actually be served by structures of the left peristriate cortex, albeit different from the ones vital for the reading process, that is portions of primary and association visual areas left intact by the lesion which produced alexia. Such structures receive visual input from the right visual system via whatever fibers have been preserved in the callosum, or else directly from the left visual system (if the patient has an intact field or a partial field defect only) but project to the posterior temporal and inferior parietal lobe via pathways which are different from those which serve reading. The case of Greenblatt (1973) supports this hypothesis. He demonstrated how in his patient *with* alexia but *without* neither color anomia nor hemianopia, the lesion had spared most of the occipital cortex, while all callosal connections had been severed at the level of the forceps major.

The significance of the dorsal splenial lesion for the argument on color anomia is further diminished, though by no means definitively so, by the findings in Benson's patient with alexia, color anomia and prosopagnosia (the lesion of the splenium was only partial also, sparing the dorsal aspect, whose intactness might have secured color naming) (Benson et al., 1974), or in Déjerine's original patient (whose callosal lesion was also ventral only), and finally by the finding of color anomia in a patient in whom the splenium was thoroughly intact (Mohr, 1971; his patient had color anomia but not alexia, and the lesions were confined to the left lateral geniculate, the white matter underlying the left lingual gyrus, the left hippocampus and parahippocampal gyrus, left fornix, left mammillary body and some left thalamic nuclei). The splenium, tapetum and forceps major were intact and so were the visual radiations and most of the occipital cortex and its underlying white matter. The inferior outflow of the occipital cortex was entirely preserved). But it must be pointed out that we have some reservations towards the notion of functional lamination of the splenium, only as it pertains to color anomia since we are convinced that as the callosal outflow diverges and courses into each hemisphere (e.g. coursing upward to arch over the lateral ventricle or caudalward to drape the medial wall of the lateral ventricle) its separate components, with separate cortical destinations may indeed perform different functions. On the other hand we have little doubt that color anomia is separable from alexia, both as a behavioral phenomenon and in terms of underlying disturbed anatomy.

Our observations in subjects with severe color anomia lead us to believe that there too, different steps of a process are being dissociated as a result of the lesion, and that we are not dealing with a singular form of functional compromise. In fact, if the color stimulus is kept constant but the testing procedure varied, patients perform in remarkably different ways. Not only do they perceive color in such a way that allows adequate matching and hue grading, but they also are able to match a color with the colorless representation of an object that generally carries it, if the task is maintained at a strictly non-verbal level. And though specific naming of colors is impaired, we found that naming of certain atributes of color is normal and so is color identification on the basis of those names. An example: patients will be able to say if colors are "light" or "dark", or sort colors that are "joyful" or "sad". This means that if the word being matched with the color has a larger semantic field than that of the specific name of a color, the patient's color anomia is overcome (Damasio, McKee, Damasio, 1979).

There is some anatomophysiological support for the behavioral distinctiveness of color anomia. Zeki (1973; 1976) has recently shown in a series of interesting experiments in the Rhesus monkey, that color is processed such as other features of visual information, in a cascade of inter-connected operators. Operators which process color do not process features such as lines or angles or depth, and have different levels of specialization in their tasks. Hence, analysis of color and of form occur separately. For instance, in the Rhesus monkey, area 17 has a small amount of cells capable of responding to color stimuli. In areas 18 and 19, no cell responds to color at all. But out of the striate belt, in the prestriate region located in the lunate sulcus and in what is designated the fourth visual area (V4), a region has been identified that not only responds solely to color but does so with a marked partitioning of which subregion responds to which color. Since all visual input of that hemisphere in the callosotomized animal has arrived in area 17 to start with, a pathway has had to transfer visual information to this area V4, a pathway that most probably travelled beneath areas 18 and 19. Further forward, out of the lunate sulcus, in the most posterior region of the superior temporal sulcus, cells will respond to color but in a different fashion, with all columns responding to more than one color and to other visual features associated to color as well. The physiological implication seems clear: as might have been expected, the nervous system has a different apparatus to process different features of stimuli. The cortical units and subserving pathways processing the complex lines which make up a letter, are not the same which handle the changes of wave length that distinguish colors.

In terms of our discussion of the anatomy of color anomia, Zeki's work suggests that alexia and color anomia can be produced by different lesions and permits some conjectures: We would suggest that lesions placed in V4 will most likely lead to the phenomena of achromatopsia, that lesions placed anteriorly to the human area V4 may lead to color anomia, and that lesions further anteriorly, that is, in multimodal association areas of the human lower parietal lobule, will be associated with aphasic misnaming not restricted to colors. Evidence from human cases supports these hypotheses. Patients with pure achromatopsia (without associated prosopagnosia) generally have strictly occipital lesions located in the lower portion of the visual association cortex (see Damasio, et al., 1980, in press), while patients with aphasic misnaming commonly have lesions in the peri-sylvian region and names of colors as well as other lexical items can be improperly utilized.

In summary, recent advances in the anatomy of pure alexia and of color anomia consist of: (a) partially separating the anatomical mechanisms responsible for pure alexia and for color anomia; (b) suggesting that dysfunction of the ventral outflow of peristriate structures is of possible importance for the production of reading disturbances; (c) demonstrating the importance of damage to subcortical left occipital structures which can be the only pathological correlate of alexia.

The evidence suggests that (a) alexia or color anomia is the result of damage not to a single main pathway but to one or more of several pertinent pathways linking a chain of processors, (b) the chain of processors and pathways which relates to color vision and color naming is, for the most part, independent from the one subtending reading.

References

Ajax, E. T.: Alexia without agraphia and the inferior splenium. Neurology 27: 685, 1977.

Benson, D. F., Segarra, J. & Albert, M. L.: Visual agnosia-prosopagnosia. A clinico-pathologic correlation. Arch Neurol 30: 307, 1974.

Brissaud, E.: Cécité verbale sans aphasie ni agraphie. Rev Neurol 8: 757, 1900.

Cumming, W. J. K., Hurwitz, L. J. & Perl, N. T.: A study of a patient who had alexia without agraphia. J Neurol Neurosurg Psychiat 33: 34, 1970.

Damasio, A. R., McKee, J. & Damasio, H.: Determinants of performance in color anomia. Brain Lang 7: 74, 1979.

Damasio, A., Yamada, T., Damasio, H., Corbett, J. & McKee, J.: Central achromatopsia: Behavioral, anatomical, and physiological aspects. Neurology, 1980 (in press).

Déjerine, J.: Contribution à l'étude anatomo-pathologique et clinique des différentes variétés de cécité verbale. Mém Soc Biol 4: 61, 1892.

Foix, C. & Hillemand, P.: Rôle vraisemblable du splénium dans la pathogénie de l'alexie pure par lésion de la cérébrale postérieure. Bull Mém Soc Méd Hôp (Paris) 49: 393, 1925.

Geschwind, N. & Fusillo, M.: Color-naming defects in association with alexia. Arch Neuro 15: 137, 1966.

Greenblatt, S. H.: Alexia without agraphia or hemianopsia. Anatomical analysis of an autopsied case. Brain 96: 307, 1973.

Greenblatt, S. H.: Subangular alexia without agraphia or hemianopsia. Brain Lang 2: 229, 1976.

Mohr, J. P., Leicester, J., Stoddard, L. T. & Sidman, M.: Right hemianopia with memory and color deficits in circumscribed left posterior cerebral artery territory infarction. Neurology 21: 1104, 1971.

Zeki, S. M.: Color coding in Rhesus monkey prestriate cortex. Brain Res 53: 422, 1973.

Zeki, S. M. & Sandeman, D. R.: Combined anatomical and electrophysiological studies on the boundary between the second and third visual areas of the Rhesus monkey cortex. Proc R Soc Med (London) B 194: 555, 1976.

Neurophysiological speech timing

KEITH KNOX AND INGRID BRAMINDER

At the Hixon Symposium, Lashley (27) remarked that he had devoted so much time to discussion of the problem of syntax, not only because language is one of the most important products of human cerebral activity, but also because the problems raised by the organization of language seemed to him to be characteristic of almost all other cerebral activity. There is a series of hierarchies of organization: the order of vocal movements in pronouncing the word, the order of words in the sentence, the order of sentences in the paragraph, the rational order of paragraphs in a discourse. Not only speech, but all skilled acts seem to involve the same problems of serial ordering, even down to the temporal coordination of muscular contractions in such a movement as reaching and grasping.

Discussion

In an inventory of 36 consonant-vowel-consonant monosyllables, MacNeilage & DeClerk (29) found some aspect of every phoneme to differ with the identity of the previous phoneme, and almost every phoneme differed in some respect depending on the one following. Each phoneme has a constellation of articulatory demands and it therefore seems reasonable that one or other aspect of each of the 44 phonemes of English, a figure from Denes (11), will vary depending on which of the 20 or so possible phonemes precedes or follows it. This infers a total of approximately 17,000 differing articulatory demands for all the various phonemes, if no account is taken of the effects of stress, speaking rate, segmentation, emotional content and phonological context. These effects are well known, however, to lend enormous variability to the acoustic correlates of a given phoneme.

All information carrying functions that are processed, transmitted and used for attaining an objective, necessarily possess the characteristic that they are not subject to precise prediction. The fluctuations of messages and noise as functions of time are extremely complex and have underlying causes which are not completely understood, with the result that no simple laws are available to exactly describe their behavior. The formation of speech waves is one example of a highly complex process which is not governed by simple laws. The purpose of speech is to transmit information and it must therefore have the characteristic that its variation as time passes cannot be predicted exactly by the listener.

Address to the "International Symposium on Aphasia" Gothenburg, Sweden, September 5–8, 1977.

SPEECH PRODUCTION ⟶ HIGHLY VARIABLE

PREDICTION OF SPEECH ⟶ IMPOSSIBLE
Fig. 1

COGNITIVE ACTIVITY ⟶ COGNITIVE
                      COMPETENCE
                    ✚ PSYCHOLOGY

LEARNED KNOWLEDGE ⟶ CONCEPT
                  ✚ HOW TO USE IT

INTUITIONS ⟶ RECURSIVE PROCEDURE
Fig. 2

DISCRIMINABILITY OF TONAL SIGNALS
⟶ DEPENDS ON ΔF x ΔT

NOT ΔF OR ΔT INDIVIDUALLY.........

BUT THE PRODUCT ΔF x ΔT
Fig. 3

It is true that at times a word or two, or even a short sequence of words, is predictable because of the rules of grammar or the occurrence of common phrases and idioms, but precise prediction is impossible. If speech could be determined exactly and completely it could not convey information. During any interval of time, however, a set of possible values exists upon which a message can be based and understood (28).

As a first look round we can say that Pylyshyn (41) suggests that a general theory of cognition should account for the structure which, with the other kinds of psychological evidence, is the output of a theory of competence. The exact form of the theory of competence, he says, should not concern us too much. It seems clear that among what we learn when we acquire certain knowledge is not only a conceptual structure, but also what might be thought of as an implicit manual on the way these concepts are to be used, and on how instances are to be assigned to them. The critical problem is to develop sound methods for tapping people's intuitions about all aspects of their cognitive function.

Basic to the notion of competence is the belief that a procedure, or a set of implicit rules, underlies such intuitions. Pylyshyn conceives this as a structure which is constructed anew each time a stimulus is encountered. To carry out this procedure, the stimulus must be analyzed into its constituent parts and relationships, and then reconstructed on the basis of this analysis. If we are to have a formal theory, Pylyshyn observes, the necessity of a finite description

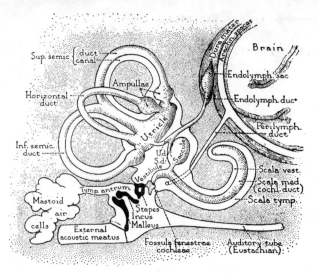

Fig. 3A. General relationships of parts of the internal and middle ear and the external auditory meatus. Diagrammatic. U.d., utricular duct; S.d., saccular duct. From Bast & Anson (1), p. 11.

forces us to characterize any concept in terms of a procedure which operates on a finite set of primitives. In linguistics none of these primitives are empirical, in the sense of being simple physical features. There is no known instrument that will identify a particular phoneme from a corresponding fragment of an acoustical waveform, much less a morpheme or a formative.

Some properties of human hearing

From experiments with human subjects, Divenyi & Danner (12) observed that for a set of noise-burst markers against a quiet background, the discriminability of a time interval has been seen to suffer to a great extent, only when less than about 25 msec and when one of two conditions was severely violated. These are (*a*) if the two signals marking the interval are not clearly audible, and (*b*) if the two signals differ excessively in their spectra.

Divenyi & Danner also noted some tendency for the bandwidth of the noise-burst markers to influence time discrimination at base intervals shorter than 30 msec, which is important in suggesting that the efficiency of the auditory signal to mark time is inversely related to the extent of short-term fluctuations in its power. This has been further confirmed by subsequent data. Divenyi & Danner came to the conclusion that the perceptual system breaks up sequential auditory information into separate streams segregated on the basis of their spectral coherence. Reception of temporal information across these streams is severely degraded.

Saprykin & Belov (45) demonstrated experimentally that for a stable frequency of false indications, human auditory perception of tonal signals depends

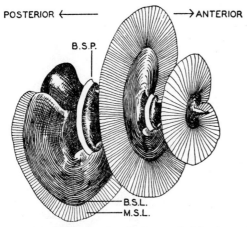

POSTERIOR ←——————   ——→ANTERIOR

B.S.P.

B.S.L.
M.S.L.

Fig. 4. Modiolus, showing the bony spiral lamina and the membranous spiral lamina (basal membrane). Right ear; viewed from lateral and slightly anterior position. The bony spiral lamina is broad in the basal and narrow in the apical turn. The membranous spiral lamina is narrow in the basal and broad in the apical turn. Only the anchorage of the bony spiral partition to the modiolus is shown. B.S.L., bony spiral lamina; B.S.P., bony spiral partition; M.S.L., membranous spiral lamina. From Bast & Anson (1), p. 93.

on the level of background noise, with frequency and duration of the signal as determining parameters. Saprykin & Sagal (46) showed that in threshold perception, the probability of correct detection of a signal depended on the product of frequency and duration and not on either separately, signifying that efficiency of threshold perception is determined by the number of waves of the harmonic signal. Samoilova & Zaitseva (44) further demonstrated that for recognition of short durations, signal processing does not cease at the moment of switching off the signal.

A proposal for the mechanism of the cochlea

Naftalin (36) hypothesizes a model in which the overall internal design of the cochlea carries out a Fourier analysis of the acoustical waveform. He stresses that the human cochlea reaches adult size and geometry by the sixth month of fetal life, after which there is no further growth (1). Naftalin's crucial point is that fixed size and unchanging geometry imply that any frequency analysis carried out by the bony labyrinth would retain its validity from birth to old age. It was established by Naftalin et al. (34) that the tectorial membrane is composed largely of a protein of the keratin-fibrinogen group and has a substantially different ionic character from endolymph and perilymph.

The tectorial membrane is in fact a gel. Since this gel is constituted upwards of 95 % of "structured water", the tectorial membrane is highly sensitive to changes in hydration. The properties of gels are of major interest here. Gels are viscoelastic, and to vibration they show a modulus of rigidity and behave as lattice-structured solids. The velocity of sound in a number of gels was measured

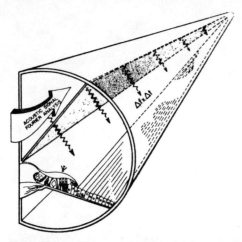

Fig. 5. The cochlea as an interface joining a continuous line capable of transmitting all frequencies and a lattice 'permitting' transmission only of defined values. The acoustic signal propagates up the scala vestibuli (which is a continuous line) and undergoes a Fourier analysis to yield Gabor (16) units of $\Delta f \cdot \Delta t$. $\Delta f \cdot \Delta t$ seeks a value Ψ in the latice, $A \cos 2 \Pi (\sqrt{t} - a\chi)$, which accepts the Gabor units. Ψ is defined by the points forming the structure of the lattice of the tectorial membrane and is continuously variable in the longitudinal direction. From Naftalin (36), p. 40.

by Naftalin & Jones (35). One of these gels was a protein of the fibrinogen group, similar in many respects to tectorial membrane. To give an example, a frequency of 1 kHz has a wavelength of 1.5 m in water, which contracts to just 5 mm in the gel.

Naftalin (36) proposed a model (37) of the cochlea in which the overall internal design of the bony labyrinth carries out a Fourier analysis of the incoming acoustic waveform, based on irreducible spectral units of frequency and duration (4, 16). These compression-rarifaction wavepackets affect the state of hydration of a restricted portion of the tectorial membrane and thereby influence the degree of complexing of the relatively loosely held magnesium known to be present there, possibly chelated (60). Naftalin makes the particularly important point that the trigger action of the magnesium ion in a charged membrane will be related quantitatively to the incoming acoustic energy. Thus the number of magnesium triggers activated will provide a quantitatively related number of signals to the hair cells (13, 60).

Vertebrate neurology, patterning and learning

Bentley (2) has shown the song of the male field cricket to be timed according to genetic rules. In the nervous system of male crickets, central pattern generators were demonstrated to produce the temporal characteristics of the male call (3). The synchronicity of the female is also genetically determined, although Hoy et al. (24) were unable to establish the precise physiological basis of female

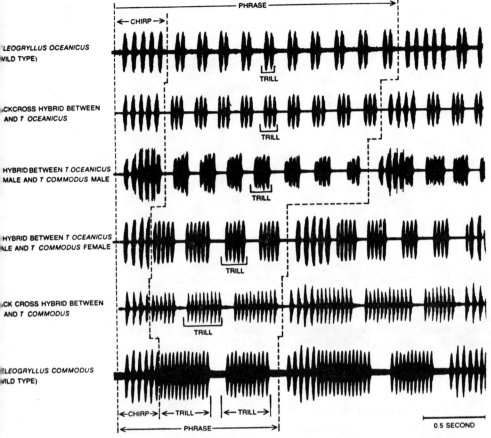

Fig. 6. Song patterns of hybrid crickets shift systematically in proportion to the ratios of the different wild-type genes inherited by the individual. These records show the song patterns of two cricket species and their hybrids. The records are aligned so that a complete phrase of the song starts at the left; each phrase consists of a chirp followed by two or more trills. The phrase of *T. oceanicus* (top) is not only much longer than the phrase of *T. commodus* (bottom) but also distinctively different. In each of the last three patterns the first trill is fused to the chirp. The F1, or first generation hybrids of these two species produced the third and fourth traces. Again they are quite different depending on which species served as the male parent and which as the female parent. The second and fifth traces were produced by backcrosses between the two different F1 hybrids and members of the parental species. From Bentley & Hoy (3), p. 40.

sensitivity to temporal patterning. This work on crickets supplies experimental support for the idea that species-specific auditory templates and feature detectors which require particular patterns of auditory input may well be important.

Weakly electric fish of the *Eigenmannia virescens* species emit an alternating field of 200–500 Hz fundamental frequency with their electric organ. Electroreceptors in the skin detect patterns of signals returning from the environment, and data from Feng & Bullock (15) suggest that the electroreceptors are used

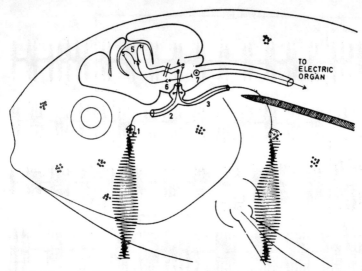

Fig. 7. Schematic diagram of the major brain centers and pathways involved in the "jamming avoidance response" in *Eigenmannia*. Information from electroreceptors (1) reaches the brain via the anterior (2) and posterior (3) branch of the anterior lateral line nerve. The first relay is the posterior lateral line lobe of the medulla (4). After crossing, the lemniscal fibers enter the torus semicircularis of the mesencephalon (5). After steps of specific integration in the torus, neurons make connections with the pacemaker in the medulla (7) via a hypothetical relay in the reticular formation (6). From Scheich (47), p. 187.

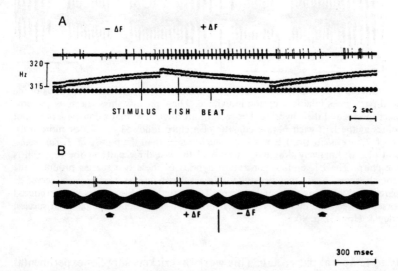

Fig. 8. The "*P*-system Δ*F*-decoder" neuron, Δ*Fp*. A simultaneous recording of the electric organ frequency during a frequency clamp and of the Δ*Fp* neuron in the midbrain. Upper trace: neuronal discharges. Two middle traces: DC equivalents of the fish and of the stimulus frequencies. The stimulus changes every 8 sec from 3 Hz below ($-\Delta F$) to the same amount above the fish's frequency ($+\Delta F$) or vice versa. Lower trace: beat envelope of the two signals. The neuron, which fires only occasionally during $-\Delta F$, gives regular bursts of activity during $+\Delta F$, synchronous with the beat cycle. Figure B shows the different phase relationship of the spike bursts to the beat cycle during $+$ and $-\Delta F$ on a faster time scale. From Scheich (49), p. 248.

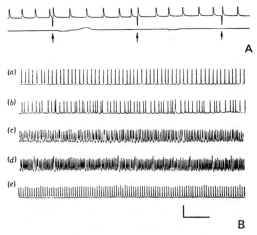

Fig. 9. (A) Intracellularly recorded e.j.ps from AAdC muscle showing resetting of the interval in a train of discharges by interpolation of a single extra impulse antidromically elicited by peripheral nerve stimulation. Time marks on the lower trace = 1 sec.

(B) Pacemaker change during learning. Effects of uplearning on pacemaker frequency of AAdC neurone. Intracellularly recorded muscle e.j.ps (*a*) after the first infusion of saline had blocked all reflex activity. Note the regularity of the discharge. (*b*) After return to normal saline and restoration of reflexes the discharge is irregular, but has a similar mean frequency. (*c*) After a first period of computer-controlled up-training. (*d*) After a second period of computer-controlled up-training. (*e*) Following a second infusion of saline. The discharge is again highly regular and it is evident that the mean frequency has been doubled. Calibrations: vertical 10 mV, horizontal 1 sec. From Woollacott & Hoyle (58), pp. 401 and 406.

to discriminate the equivalent impedance and spatial orientation of objects in the surroundings of the fish.

The same set of electroreceptors detect electric organ discharge fields from neighboring fish. Scheich (47, 48, 49) investigated electric fish jamming avoidance responses, in which avoidance tactics to a foreign frequency were examined. An electric fish of the *Eigenmannia virescens* species will detect a signal from another fish and move its own frequency away within about half a cycle. Scheich discovered that the patterns in the neuronal system of the lateral line nerve indicated the use of time domain analysis to examine beats between the two frequencies. This was interesting, but it did not explain the precision and speed of the normal behavior of the fish.

Scheich proceeded further and observed neuron patterns in the posterior lobe of the medulla and in the torus semicircularis of the midbrain. He was not able to determine precisely how it was achieved, but he was able to demonstrate with certainty, that there was a change in the demodulation pattern to a simple frequency code, with extremely fine detector precision indeed. Scheich was not able to show that the torus was a pacemaker, but his results did show that the torus played a key role in the motor control of the pacemaker.

Woollacott & Hoyle (58) examined locusts of the species *Schistocerca gregaria* and were able to demonstrate to an exceedingly high level of confi-

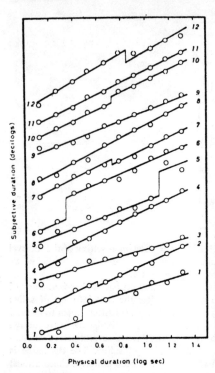

Fig. 10. Linear plots obtained for twelve subjects when magnitude estimates were plotted against stimulus durations on loglog coordinates. This shows that subjects give magnitude estimates which follow a power function. Eisler had already shown that the psychophysical function for ratio settings is a power function. Breaks in the curves depend on whether the scale unit, the subjective zero, or both, are different for the different segments. From Eisler (14), p. 443.

dence indeed that the anterior adductor of the coxa (AAdC) functioned as a pacemaker. They were furthermore able to demonstrate that a number of shock avoidance tactics were *learned* by the locust by use of the pacemaker. Woollacott & Hoyle state confidently that their results provide direct evidence, the first of which they are cognizant, of pacemaker change as a physiological event underlying a learning phenomenon. For purposes of this presentation, we wish to implicate this technique as a potential cognitive mechanism of the greatest generality.

Is there a human pacemaker?

Measurements of subjective time duration carried out by Sagal & Bagrova (43) and Eisler (14) for human subjects, seem to finally establish that subjective

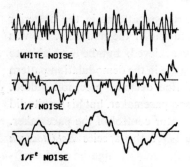

Fig. 11. Samples of white noise, $1/f$ noise and $1/f^2$ noise. From Voss & Clarke (56), fig. 1.

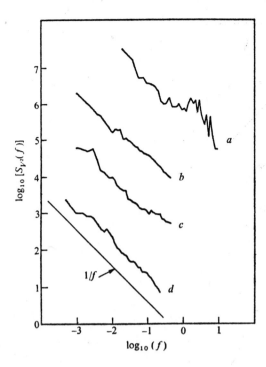

Fig. 12. Loudness fluctuation spectra, $S_v2(f)$ versus f for: (*a*) Scott Joplin piano rags, (*b*) classical radio station, (*c*) rock radio station, (*d*) news and talk radio station. From Voss & Clarke (56), fig. 4.

time follows a power function. Sagal & Bagrova note the following. "It may be assumed that the higher nervous activity acts as a complex adaptive system, with variable characteristics of activity. It is natural to represent the sensory space of the reflexion as a space with a variable metric. In conditions of optimal activity, the sensory metric becomes the simple linear function of the imposed metric of the stimuli."

We can go further and suggest that a difference between subjective time and mechanically measured time, is probably an indication that a message is being competently transmitted and understood. This signifies a high likelihood of direct correlation between the relation of subjective and mechanically measured time, with what is known as a subject's "tactics of attention". It seems intuitively reasonable to assume that the aesthetics of communication are to be discovered in the efficiency of communication brought about by this method of focusing, which is the subjective time experience.

Some long-term spectral properties of speech

The power spectrum is an extremely useful way of characterizing the average behavior of any quantity which varies with time. This method is most often used for the analysis of random signals, or "noise", but for many physical quantities the power spectrum varies approximately as the inverse of frequency over many decades of frequency. This spectrum is known as "1/f-like".

10 – 804513 *Aphasia*

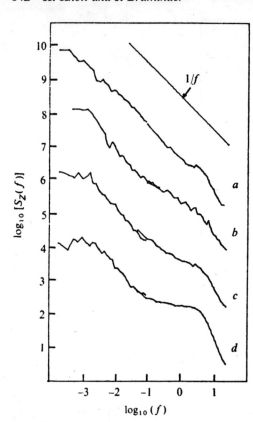

Fig. 12A. Power spectra of pitch fluctuations $S_z(f)$ versus f for: (*a*) classical radio station, (*b*) jazz & blues radio station. (*c*) rock radio station, (*d*) news and talk radio station. From Voss & Clarke (56), fig. 5.

Vacuum tubes (26), carbon resistors (7), semiconductors (59), continuous (10, 23) or discontinuous (57) metal film, ionic solutions (21), films at the super-conducting transition (9), Josephson junctions (8), nerve membranes (54), sunspot activity (31) and the flood levels of the River Nile (31), all exhibit "$1/f$-like" fluctations (56). The $1/f$ spectrum implies that some correlation exists in these fluctuating quantities over all time scales corresponding to the frequency range for which the power spectrum is "$1/f$-like".

As a result of carrying out long-term measurements of music and speech, Voss & Clarke (55) showed that the power spectra of the loudness fluctuations for many musical selections and for English speech down to a frequency of 5×10^{-4} Hz, were also "$1/f$-like". The pitch fluctuations of music were also shown to have a "$1/f$-like" power spectrum at frequencies down to the inverse of the length of the piece. Pitch fluctuations of English speech behave quite differently and show a single characteristic time, with a power spectrum that is "white" below about 3 Hz and which falls off as $1/f^2$ down to about 3 Hz. Voss & Clarke established by this means that the average length of an individual speech sound, over a long term, is equivalent to approximately 0.1 sec. This is a very important result, which may be interpreted as direct evidence for a measure of average constancy in speech rate. Voss & Clarke explain that the

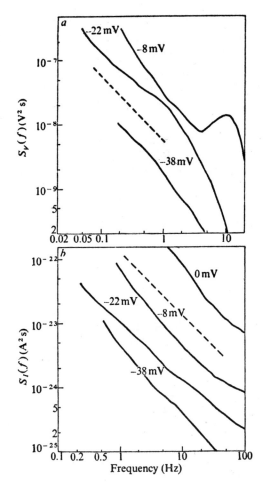

Fig. 13. Power spectra of stationary membrane noise at various membrane potentials. Standard solution at 19°C. (a) Noise voltage spectra $S_v(f)$, measured under current clamp. Electronic noise negligible. (b) Noise current spectra $S_i(f)$, measured under voltage clamp. Electronic noise negligible up to about 50 Hz, but exceeding membrane noise above 100 Hz. Note the difference in frequency scale. Dashed lines represent slope -1. Spectra are related according to $S_v(f) = S_i(f)/|Z_m(f)|^2$. From Moolenaar et al. (33), p. 345.

pitches of the individual speech sounds are unrelated for normal English speech, since the ideas are not related to the pitches but to the meanings attached to the syllables.

Some properties of "$1/f$-like" distributions

It can be assumed that for the power spectra of loudness fluctuations, a long-term "$1/f$-like" distribution is an important property of at least English speech. It is reasonable therefore to look more closely into what this means. Hooge (22) carried out a survey of physical occurrence of "$1/f$-like" noise and decided tentatively that the fluctuations were a result of electron mobility, rather than of electron number. Brophy (6) experimentally investigated the statistics of a "$1/f$-like" distribution in a carbon resistor, and discovered that a variance-of-variance existed in the fluctuations. Brophy described his findings as "noisy noise"; a non-stationary fluctuation in some weaker form of conditional stationarity. Over the years a number of mathematical models have been proposed for "1/f-like" noise distributions (19, 20, 30, 38, 39, 50, 51) but to date no physical basis is known for any of them. It was certainly an embarrassment for progress in physiology to discover (54) that vertebrate nerve membranes and nerve fibers exhibited "1/f-like" noise properties (53).

This matter became extremely serious when Moolenaar et al. (33) demonstrated that the "1/f-like" noise fluctuations of a resting membrane could be disturbed and cause the membrane to operate. It was precisely by this means that Moolenaar and his coworkers were able to observe the ciliated protozoan, *Paramecium*, swimming backwards. Their report provided the first experimental evidence for a connection between membrane "1/f-like" noise and simple behavioral effects in a living organism.

Two diagnostic techniques

The long-term average length of an individual speech sound in English was found by Voss & Clarke (55) to be roughly 0.1 sec. Jaffe et al. (25) observe that despite wide variations in methods of assessing speech rate, there is general agreement about the proposition that when human communication is pathological the *range* of speech rates is greater than would be expected from that same group of patients under normal conditions.

This range of speech rates seems more in the nature of a band with upper and lower limits. The diagnostic categories of stuttering-cluttering disorders, aphasias, Parkinson disorders and manic-depressive psychosis, occasion speech rates both higher and lower than the norm. In some of these categories the distribution of patient's speech rate is clearly bimodal, and in some categories a given patient oscillates between modes on repeated testing. This suggests that the unimodal distribution of speech rates seen in normal populations is the outcome of some homeostatic mechanism, which maintains an optimum rate and counteracts extreme deviations in either direction. Neurophysiological evidence for the inherent bimodality in neural control of speech rate derives from stimulation of the ventrolateral nucleus of the thalamus in the dominant hemisphere during neurosurgical procedures (5). Such stimulation may produce either arrest of speech, or an uncontrollably rapid rate (18).

Middle evoked electroencephalic responses to sound, with latencies of 8–50 msec duration, have been examined in infants by McRandle et al. (32). In a complex spectrum of responses, clearly identifiable middle evoked components were found with ease 36 to 72 hours after birth in all ten of a group of human neonates. McRandle et al. note that middle evoked components appear in infants with the same regularity as they do in adults. This finding suggests that the neutral substrate is sufficiently mature in the early perinatal period to produce adult-like waveforms. These workers believe that the auditory responses which they found reflect primary auditory system activity, with a

The suggestion is made that the coherence which underlies Lashley's (27) series of hierarchies of language organization, depends on a continuing statistical description of any ensemble pattern of speech.

The "1/f-like" loudness spectrum of speech infers particular kinds of constraints on the growth and decay of the spectral energy associated with individual elements within any ensemble.

Fig. 14

stability and regularity of latency that argues a contribution for their genesis along the direct lemniscal pathway. McRandle et al. also note that significant aberrations of amplitude and waveform occur in these responses from some adult aphasics and they encourage the use of their technique in the assessment of central nervous system dysfunction.

Summary and conclusions

Based on the evidence presented here, we would like most strongly to urge efforts aimed at correlating long samples of instantaneous loudness spectra, taken from human speech in a variety of languages, with regularities of recursiveness such as those described by Pylyshyn (41) in his examination of the factors underlying competence.

Pylyshyn's theory takes the form of a formal mechanism which computes a certain recursive function. This function consists of the enumeration of a set of sequences of behavior called the possible idealized, or normative behaviors, together with two kinds of structural description. The first of Pylyshyn's structural descriptions relates various elements within a behavioral sequence. The second relates such elements and sequences to other elements and sequences in the set of possible idealized behaviors. Due to the recursive nature of this function, there are an unlimited number of ways of describing competence. All are formally equivalent, and the precise form is determined by principles of internal coherence and economy.

Pylyshyn's form of expression is merely another way of describing Lashley's (27) series of hierarchies of language organization: the order of vocal movements in pronouncing the word, the order of words in the sentence, the order of sentences in the paragraph, the rational order of paragraphs in a discourse.

Two possible ways can be distinguished for going about the practical work of seeking correlations. Either the prior probability distribution may be postulated (17, 40) and confirmed or refuted on the basis of evidential data. Or it is sometimes possible to determine certain properties of an unknown distribution by deriving suitable functions from the marginal deviations of the distribution (42). Language researchers have succeeded in amassing a very substantial body of evidence of particular kinds of human speech variability in production, and it would be at least interesting to know if these different areas of speech variability carry detectable correlative regularities in long samples of their loudness fluctuations. New theoretical illustrations of classes of "1/f-like" noise will also, of course, be welcome.

Finally, it seems clear that human speech is quite capable of providing significant additional knowledge about "1/f-like" distributions, which could be of potential value to progress in physiology, biochemistry, psycholinguistics, and areas of physics alike.

References

1. Bast, T. H. & Anson, B. J.: The temporal bone and the ear. Thomas, Springfield, 1949.
2. Bentley, D. R.: Intracellular activity in cricket neurons during the generation of song patterns. Z Vgl Physiol 62: 267, 1969.
3. Bentley, D. R. & Hoy, R. R.: The neurobiology of cricket song. Sc Am 231: 34, 1974.
4. Billings, A. R. & Scolaro, A. B.: The Gabor compression-expansion system using non-Gaussian windows and its application to television coding and decoding. IEEE Trans Inf Theory IT-22: 174, 1976.
5. Botez, M. I. & Barbeau, A.: The role of subcortical structures and particularly of the thalamus, in the mechanisms of speech and language. Int J Neurol 8: 300, 1971.
6. Brophy, J. J.: Statistics of 1/f noise. Phys Rev 166: 827, 1968.
7. Christensen, C. J. & Pearson, G. L.: Spontaneous resistance fluctuations in carbon microphones and other granular resistances. Bell Syst Tech J 15: 197, 1936.
8. Clarke, J. & Hawkins, G.: Low frequency noise in Josephson junctions. IEEE Trans on Magnetics MAG-11: 841, 1975.
9. Clarke, J. & Hsiang, T. Y.: Low frequency noise in tin films at the superconducting transition. Phys Rev Lett 34: 1217, 1975.
10. Clarke, J. & Voss, R. F.: 1/f noise from thermal fluctuations in metal films. Phys Rev Lett 33: 24, 1974.
11. Denes, P. B.: On the statistics of spoken English. J Acoust Soc Am 35: 892, 1963.
12. Divenyi, P. L. & Danner, W. F.: Discrimination of time intervals marked by brief acoustic pulses of various intensities and spectra. Perc Psychophys 21: 125, 1977.
13. Eigen, M. & Hammes, G. C.: Elementary steps in enzyme reactions. In: Advances in Enzymology, vol. 25 (ed. F. F. Nord), pp. 1–38. Wiley-Interscience, New York, 1963.
14. Eisler, H.: Subjective duration and psychophysics. Psych Rev 82: 429, 1975.
15. Feng, A. S. & Bullock, T. H.: Neuronal mechanisms for object discrimination in the weakly electric fish Eigenmannia virescens. J Exp Biol 66: 141, 1977.
16. Gabor, D.: Theory of communication. J Inst Elect Engr 93: 429, 1946.
17. Gardner, W. A. & Franks, L. E.: Characterization of cyclostationary random signal processes. IEEE Trans Inf Theory IT-21: 4, 1975.
18. Guiot, G., Herzog, E., Roudot, P. & Molina, P.: Arrest or acceleration of speech evoked by thalamic stimulation in the course of stereotaxic procedures for Parkinsonism. Brain 84: 363, 1961.

19. Halford, D.: A general mechanical model for $/f/^{-\alpha}$ spectral density random noise, with special reference to flicker noise $/f/^{-1}$. Proc IEEE 56: 251, 1968.
20. Heiden, C.: Power spectrum of stochastic pulse sequences with correlation between the pulse parameters. Phys Rev 188: 319, 1969.
21. Hooge, F. N.: $1/f$ noise in the conductance of ions in aqueous solutions. Phys Lett 33 A: 169, 1970.
22. Hooge, F. N.: Discussion of recent experiments on $1/f$ noise. Physica 60: 130, 1972.
23. Hooge, F. N. & Hoppenbrouwes, A. M. H.: $1/f$ noise in continuous thin gold films. Physica 45: 386, 1969.
24. Hoy, R. R., Hahn, J. & Paul, R. C.: Hybrid cricket auditory behavior—evidence for genetic coupling in animal communication. Science 195: 82, 1977.
25. Jaffe, J., Anderson, S. W. & Rieber, R. W.: Research and clinical approaches to disorders of speech rate. J Comm Disorders 6: 225, 1973.
26. Johnson, J. B.: The Schottky effect in low frequency circuits. Phys Rev 26: 71, 1925.
27. Lashley, K. S.: The problem of serial order in behavior. In: Cerebral Mechanisms in Behavior (ed. L. A. Jeffress), pp. 112–136. Wiley, New York, 1951.
28. Lee, Y. W.: Statistical Theory of Communication. Wiley, New York, 1960.
29. MacNeilage, P. F. & DeClerk, J. L.: On the motor control of coarticulation in CVC monosyllables. J Acoust Soc Am 45: 1217, 1969.
30. Mandelbrot, B.: Some noises with $1/f$ spectrum, a bridge between direct current and white noise. IEEE Trans Inf Theory IT-13: 289, 1967.
31. Mandelbrot, B. & Wallis, J. R.: Water Resources. RES 5: 321, 1969.
32. McRandle, C. C., Smith, M. A. & Goldstein, R.: Early averaged electroencephalic to clicks in neonates. Ann Otol Rhinol Laryng 83: 695, 1974.
33. Moolenaar, W. H., de Goede, J. & Verveen, A. A.: Membrane noise in Paramecium. Nature 260: 344, 1976.
34. Naftalin, L., Harrison, M. S. & Stephens, A.: The character of the tectorial membrane. J Laryngol Otol 78: 1061, 1964.
35. Naftalin, L. & Jones, G. P.: Propogation of acoustic waves in gels with special reference to the theory of hearing. Life Sci(I) 8: 765, 1969.
36. Naftalin, L.: The perpheral hearing mechanism—a biochemical and biological approach. Ann Otol Rhinol Laryng 85: 38, 1976.
37. Naftalin, L.: A more comprehensive exposition of the material dealt with in Naftalin (36) is scheduled to appear in Physiological Chemistry & Physics: in press. New York.
38. Offner, F. F.: $1/f$ noise in semiconductors. J Appl Phys 41: 5033, 1970.
39. Offner, F. F.: $1/f$ fluctuation in membrane potential as related to membrane theory. Biophys J 11: 123, 1971.
40. Pfaffelhuber, E.: Generalized harmonic analysis for distributions. IEEE Trans Inf Theory IT-21: 605, 1975.
41. Pylyshyn, Z. W.: The role of competence theories in cognitive psychology. J Psycholing Res 2: 21, 1974.
42. Rao, C. R.: Linear Statistical Inference and Its Applications. Wiley, New York, 1965.
43. Sagal, A. A. & Bagrova, N. D.: Construction of the natural scales of the duration of tonal sounds. Biophys 17: 941, 1972.
44. Samoilova, I. K. & Zaitseva, K. A.: Recognition of complex bound signals of different duration in sequential complex. Biophys 16: 1144, 1971.
45. Saprykin, V. A. & Belov, B. I.: Evaluation of the probability characteristics of the human auditory analyzer on perception of tonal sounds in noise. Biophys 13: 1261, 1968.

46. Saprykin, V. A. & Sagal, A. A.: Invariance of the ability to detect tonal sounds relative to the operation of compression (widening) of the signal. Biophys 17: 523, 1972.

47. Scheich, H.: Neural basis of communication in the high frequency electric fish, Eigenmannia virescens (jamming avoidance response). Part 1. Open loop experiments and the time domain concept of signal analysis. J Comp Physiol (A) 113: 181, 1977.

48. Scheich, H.: Neural basis of communication in the high frequency electric fish, Eigenmannia virescens, (jamming avoidance response). Part 2. Jammed electroreceptor neurons in the lateral line nerve. J Comp Physiol (A) 113: 207, 1977.

49. Scheich, H.: Neural basis of communication in the high frequency electric fish, Eigenmannia virescens (jamming avoidance response). Part 3. Central integration in the sensory pathway and control of the pacemaker. J Comp Physiol (A) 113: 229, 1977.

50. Teitler, S. & Osborne, M. F. M.: Phenomenological approach to low frequency electrical noise. J Appl Phys 41: 3274, 1970.

51. Tunaley, J. K. E.: Nyquist's theorem and $1/f$ noise. J Appl Phys 45: 482, 1974.

52. Tunaley, J. K. E.: A theory of $1/f$ current noise based on a random walk model. J Statist Phys 15: 149, 1976.

53. Verveen, A. A. & DeFelice, L. J.: Membrane noise. In: Progress in Biophysics, no. 28 (ed. A. J. V. Butler & D. Noble), pp. 189–265. Pergamon, Oxford, 1974.

54. Verveen, A. A. & Derksen, H. E.: Fluctuation phenomena in nerve membrane. Proc IEEE 56: 906, 1968.

55. Voss, R. F. & Clarke, J.: $1/f$ noise in music and speech. Nature 258: 317, 1975.

56. Voss, R. F. & Clarke, J.: $1/f$ noise in music: music from $1/f$ noise. Personal communication, 1977.

57. Williams, J. L. & Burdett, R. K.: Current noise in thin gold films. J Phys 2 C: 298, 1969.

58. Woollacott, M. & Hoyle, G.: Neural events underlying learning in insects—changes in pacemaker. Proc R Soc Lond (B) 195: 395, 1977.

59. van der Ziel, A.: Noise—Sources, Characterization, Measurement, p. 106. Prentice-Hall, Englewood Cliffs, 1970.

60. A "flexible molecule" with a chelating group has two dipole components, the first rigidly fixed in the molecule and the second with one or other of two equivalent positions relative to the first, and relative to the molecular axes. The relaxation time of many magnesium chelates is much greater than for chelates of the alkali metals and the other alkaline earths, and lies in the time range of 10^{-4} to 10^{-2} sec. For a discussion see (13).

Treatment of aphasia on a linguistic basis

DOROTHEA WENIGER, WALTER HUBER, FRANZ-JOSEF
STACHOWIAK AND KLAUS POECK

Introduction

In most neuropsychological centres aphasia is considered mainly a research
problem and the therapeutic aspect of the disorder is given little consideration.
This is rather surprising because aphasia is one of the most frequently observed syndromes in neurology. About 85 % of all patients with cerebrovascular accidents have a vascular insufficiency in the territory of one of the
carotid arteries. The left and the right carotid arteries are affected with the
same frequency. This means that about 40 % of all CVAs occur in the left
hemisphere. Considering the anatomy of cerebral vascularization, it is
reasonable to assume that most patients with left-sided brain damage due to a
CVA are aphasic. Not in all cases of aphasia, however, will speech therapy
be necessary; a certain percentage of patients do not survive the CVA,
others have a spontaneous recovery. According to our experience half of the
patients with a left hemispheric stroke need speech therapy. The number of
these patients is considerable. But the belief is still widespread that recovery
from aphasia is largely a matter of chance and takes place spontaneously
and that speech therapy has little more than an unspecific activating effect, serv-
ing in severe cases as a kind of psychotherapeutic aid that prevents the patient
from realizing his hopeless situation.

In those centres where aphasic patients do receive systematic speech
therapy, the regime is usually intuitive and based on the experiences with
second language learning. But everybody would agree that the situation of
someone learning a second language and of an aphasic patient is different.

Undoubtedly, aphasia therapy should be based on a precise analysis of the
linguistic deficits of the particular aphasic syndrome (5, 8, 9, 12). Although
patients with a certain aphasic syndrome are impaired in varying degrees
with regards to their deficit in different linguistic modalities, there is a
characteristic combination of symptoms constituting specific syndromes. It is
therefore possible to analyze the component deficits of a syndrome and to
design specific therapy programs that only require slight modifications for the
individual patient. These programs are not aimed at teaching the patient to
deal with certain linguistic segments—phonemes, inflectional endings, pre-
positional phrases in isolation—but rather to use again the linguistic
strategies by which words, sentences and discourse are produced (10).

In the literature there are very few reports on the effect of specific therapy in the sense outlined above. An important pilot study was done by Carol Wiegel-Crump (13) who compared the performance of agrammatic patients under two therapy conditions. Patients receiving merely conversational stimulation showed no improvement in a picture description task whereas patients that had been given programmed language therapy not only did significantly better in the same task but were able to generalize from drilled items to non-drilled items. In another therapy experiment in which patients with amnesic aphasia had to name pictures, the same author demonstrated an improvement in retrieving non-drilled items from superordinate categories drilled as well as non-drilled (14). This is again evidence that programmed language therapy leads to an improvement of linguistic abilities in the aphasic patient.

Aphasia therapy may be regarded successful if the following four stages of improvement are acquired:

— The improvement of certain linguistic abilities achieved by repeated practice must be stabilized, i.e. it must be demonstrated that the achieved improvement lasts beyond the period of therapy.
— There ought not only be an improvement with regards to the material practiced but also with regards to similarly structured non-practiced material. In other words a generalization ought to take place.
— Stabilization should also be achieved with this generalization effect.
— Therapy should lead to an improvement of spontaneous speech performance.

In the following sections we shall discuss these stages on the basis of pilot studies in which the efficacy of linguistically oriented therapy is tested.

Stabilization and generalization

Let me first turn to evidence demonstrating the stabilization and generalization of therapy effects. A fifty-nine year old teacher had a stroke which left him with a Wernicke's aphasia characterized by severe phonemic jargon and very poor auditory comprehension. He was unable to repeat and to name on confrontation. The patient's reading for understanding with regards to simple concrete nouns was relatively well preserved so that therapy could be based on written material. In the study to be reported (Huber et al., 7) the patient was given two training periods, each followed by an interval of three weeks during which no therapy was given. The first training period was 4 weeks long and the second 3 weeks long. The aim of the training program was to enable the patient to pronounce correctly all basic German consonants and important consonant clusters in simple concrete nouns. The patient had to read aloud these nouns. Various methods were applied, the most effective being Schuell's direct auditory stimulation (11). Pre- and post therapy tests were used in order to assess the patient's subsequent improvement; these

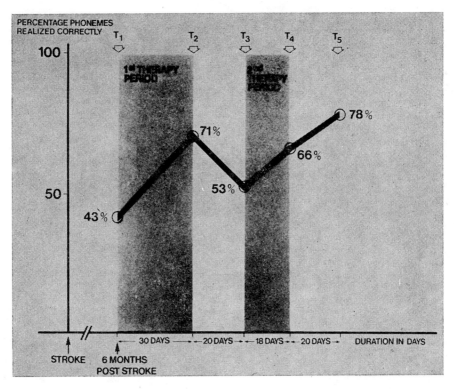

Fig. 1. Course of therapy. Rating based on control tests before and after each therapy period.

tests consisted of reading aloud same and different nouns without any assistance from the therapist. The scoring practice was the following: a point was given for each phoneme realized correctly in the right word position. As the length of the individual nouns varied, between 2 to 5 points could be obtained for a single word. Sixty words were used both in the therapy and the test situations, twenty words were only used in the test situation. Fig. 1 shows the results of the experiment.

After the first training period the patient had a gain of 28 % in his reading performance; when Wilcoxon's matched-pairs signed-ranks test was applied this difference turned out to be significant at the 0.01 level. After the first interval in which the patient received no therapy the patient's performance dropped to the pretherapy level. After the second therapy period the patient's performance rose significantly to 60 %. At the end of the second no therapy interval this level was maintained, numerically performance was even better. Here, stabilization could be observed only after the second therapy period. One could argue that the stabilization of the therapy effect was a matter of spontaneous remission. But since the experiment was run six months post stroke it seems unlikely that this was the case. That stabilization did not take place until after the second period of therapy may be due to the general

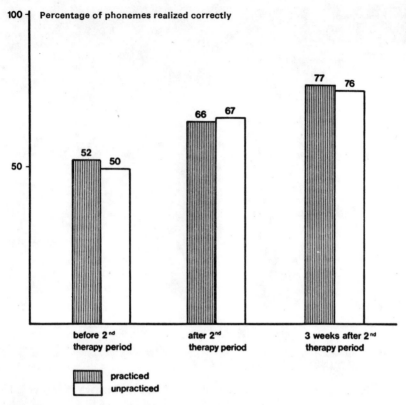

Fig. 2. Generalization and stabilization of practiced and unpracticed phonemic realization.

experience that the alternation between periods of training and no training is better suited to consolidate learning material (Foppa, 3, Carson et al., 2).

We introduced unpracticed material before and after the second training period as well as after the second period of no therapy. Interestingly enough, a similar improvement and stabilization could be observed. In other words, the patient had not only learned to read aloud sixty specific nouns but also to pronounce the basic phonemes of German as contained in these sixty nouns. Fig. 2 shows the results.

The following example is meant to illustrate stabilization and generalization on the syntactic level. A 49-year-old bank manager suffered a left hemispheric CVA which left him with a right-sided hemiplegia and Broca's aphasia, characterized mainly by severe agrammatism. After having received speech therapy for 18 months a special program was designed to treat the patient's persistent agrammatism. The patient was given 15 pictures depicting everyday situations; the task was to describe each of these pictures with a sentence. To eliminate possible lexical problems and to be able to focus on particular sentence patterns the patient was given an array of cards on which the constituents of the target sentence were printed. Before a sentence was drilled the

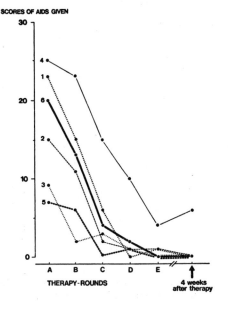

SCORES OF AIDS GIVEN

THERAPY-ROUNDS

4 weeks after therapy

Fig. 3. Improvement of syntactic performance in various modalities during and after therapy (1–6 = linguistic modalities, see text).

patient had to order these constituents. The sentences were of increasing syntactic complexity, for example:

The man is smoking a pipe
Mother is reading the book to the children

The whole set of 15 sentences was drilled in 5 separate rounds. In each round the target sentence was practiced in 6 modalities:

1. Ordering of sentence constituents (see above).
2. Correctly ordered sentence read aloud.
3. Correctly ordered sentence copied.
4. Ordered sentence written from memory.
5. Sentence written from memory read aloud.
6. Picture described orally from memory.

Scoring was based on the degree of aids the patient received from the therapist in each of the above mentioned six modalities. Two degrees, slight and strong, were distinguished. Fig. 3 shows clearly that the scores decreased considerably from one round to the next, especially in the third round.

To examine whether this improvement was not simply due to the repetiveness of the task a pre- and post therapy control test was performed. The patient was given two sets of 15 pictures, 15 of which were situationally similar to the drilled pictures, 15 of which were different. In both of these control tests the patient had to describe the pictures with a sentence. The sentences were tape-recorded, transcribed and given to 8 raters to judge. The raters did not know which of the two sentences in each pair to be com-

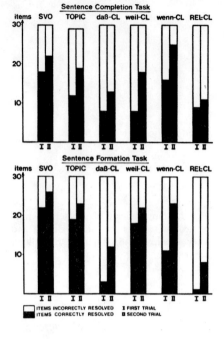

Fig. 4. Improvement in sentence completion and sentence formation tasks.

pared was produced by the patient in the pre- and post therapy control test. All raters agreed that the patient's post training performance was linguistically more adequate. This was true for both sets of stimulus pictures. Thus it is justified to conclude that the improvement generalized to non-drilled, similar items as well as different items. As in the previous experiment stabilization of the therapy effect could be demonstrated when the patient was given one round of the therapy program again four weeks after the therapy period as can be seen in Fig. 3. The degree of aids necessary remained on the low level reached in the last round of the therapy period.

Transfer of therapy effects to spontaneous language performance

So far we have given examples of how stabilization and generalization may be achieved. But of course the ultimate aim of any therapy is an improvement of spontaneous verbal communication. The degree of improvement to be expected depends on the severity and type of language disturbance. Let us illustrate this point with the case of a 23-year-old patient with developmental aphasia (6).

This case is particularly interesting because no spontaneous improvement could be reasonably expected to interfere with the effect of therapy during the experimental period. The patient was given a four weeks' intensive training program with daily therapy sessions. The training program consisted of sentence completion and sentence formation tasks in which the basic repertory

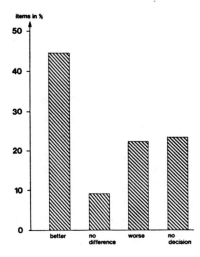

Fig. 5. Improvement in story completion as judged by 20 raters.

of German sentence patterns was drilled. Before and after the therapy period the patient was tested with material requiring the application of the same syntactic patterns but making use of different lexical material. Therapy resulted in a clear improvement of performance with regards to each task as well as with regards to each syntactic pattern.

Furthermore, we were interested in knowing whether this improvement was not only restricted to the therapy situation but could also be observed in a task comparable with spontaneous verbal communication. The patient was given 76 stories to complete. The stories all focussed on a real life situation with a high degree of familiarity. For example: An accident just happened and the police have arrived; many people crowd around. The policeman gets out of his car, looks around for the driver and asks ... (what?). In order to complete these stories different speech acts such as questions, commands, and statements must be realized. The stories were given before and after the period in which sentence patterns were drilled. The patients' responses were judged by 20 raters who did not know the patient nor whether the sentences they judged came from the test administered before or after the therapy period. The raters—medical staff, psychologists, linguists and speech therapists— had to decide which of any two responses was linguistically more adequate.

In 44.7% of the sentence pairs the raters agreed on an improvement, in contrast, 22.4% were judged less adequate. Pattern drill, in this case the training of syntactic patterns and lexical items, led to a general improvement in the use of speech acts in a task comparable to normal verbal communication.

Therapy on different linguistic levels

In the last part of this paper we should like to illustrate some linguistic aspects essential to aphasia therapy by focussing on disorders on different linguistic levels. With regards to the *phonemic level* we find disorders mainly in patients with Wernicke's, Broca's, conduction and global aphasia. We want to stress that in speaking of phonemic disorders we are restricting ourselves to only those disturbances which are aphasic in nature. We shall not speak of omission, substitution, addition, etc. which are due to cortical dysarthria and apraxia of speech. In aphasia, phonemic disorders are not only found in speech production and comprehension but also in reading and writing. This is due to the fact that in aphasia the phonemic inventory as well as the rules for combining phonemes is affected. Therefore, in aphasia therapy the linguistic function of phonemes, i.e. the differentiation of meaning in the context of words, must be trained rather than the produc-tion of isolated phonemes—which by themselves carry no meaning. In actual therapy this principle is realized by having the patient practice phonemes in the context of minimal phonemic contrast, e.g. *candle* vs.—*handle*. Such an approach requires that the semantic content of these words is made clear to the patient either by showing him a picture of the particular object or by giving him sentence frames in which only the target word fits (e.g. *he lit the ... on the Christmas tree*) (1, 4).

Basically, the procedure is the same in treating *syntactic disorders*. In agram-matism sentence patterns are reduced so that the syntactic forms which are necessary in constructing questions, commands and statements cannot be produced. However, the communicative function of these forms is preserved in comprehension.

The patient can distinguish a question from a command. Therapy can make use of this fact by having various sentence forms practiced in pragmatic contexts, i.e. the presuppositions, connotations and implications associated with situations in which specific sentences are uttered. There are various techniques with which such pragmatic contexts can be created in order to elicit the sentence forms to be practiced, e.g. story completion, picture stories, slides, video scenes.

Lexical disturbances are seen in all types of aphasia. They typically consist in word substitutions where the realized word usually has a classifica-tory or propositional relation to the target word (5). In instances of classifica-tory misnaming the word uttered belongs to the same semantic class as the target word (*goat* instead of *sheep*, *cow* instead of *horse*); propositional misnaming consists in uttering a word which refers to a situation in which the target word tends to occur (*apple* instead of *crossbow*). The consequences to be drawn for therapy are that not only the paradigmatic aspects should be practiced as is usually done by having pictures sorted according to semantic classes, but syntagmatic aspects should be practiced as well and this is best done by training words in sentences. In sentences, words impose selection restrictions on the kind of words to be combined. This is particularly important for patients with Wernicke's aphasia whose paragrammatic sen-tences are often deviant because selection restrictions are violated.

The examples which we have briefly sketched make it clear that aphasia therapy ought not be restricted to just practicing linguistic segments on single linguistic levels. In setting up therapy programs the functional connections between linguistic components are not only basic to the description of the aphasic syndrome but also for aphasia therapy. We postulate that a therapy program which is based on linguistic principles is superior to conventional methods in which only isolated phonemes, words or sentences are drilled and also to a mode of therapy by which the patient is mostly given motivation and encouragement, leaving linguistic improvement to the process of spontaneous recovery. The linguistic methods we are speaking of must be rigorous and specific, they must be derived from experiments in which the efficacy of a given method has been clearly demonstrated. The pilot studies which we report in this paper are examples of how we think such experiments should be designed.

References

1. Boller, F. & Green, E.: Comprehension in severe aphasics. Cortex 8: 382, 1972.
2. Carson, D. H., Carson, F. E. & Tikofsky, R. S.: On learning characteristics of the adult aphasic. Cortex 4: 92, 1968.
3. Foppa, K.: Lernen, Gedächtnis, Verhalten: Ergebnisse und Probleme der Lernpsychologie. Kiepenheuer & Witsch, Köln, 1965.
4. Green, E. Boller, F.: Features of auditory comprehension in severely impaired aphasics. Cortex 10: 133, 1974.
5. Huber, W., Stachowiak, F.-J., Poeck, K. & Kerschensteiner, M.: Die Wernicke Aphasie. Klinisches Bild und Überlegungen zur neurolinguistischen Struktur. J Neurol 210: 77, 1975.
6. Huber, W., Kerschensteiner, M. & Mayer, I.: Untersuchungen zur Prognose und Methode der Therapie von Entwicklingsaphasie. Nervenarzt 48: 40, 1977.
7. Huber, W., Mayer, I. & Kerschensteiner, M.: Untersuchungen zur Methode und zum Verlauf der Therapie von phonematischem Jargon bei Wernicke-Aphasie. Folia phoniat. 30: 119, 1978.
8. Kerschensteiner, M., Poeck, K., Huber, W., Stachowiak, F.-J. & Weniger, D.: Die Broca Aphasie. Klinisches Bild und Überlegungen zur neurolinguistischen Struktur. J Neurol 217: 223, 1978.
9. Poeck, K., Kerschensteiner, M., Stachowiak, F.-J. & Huber, W.: Die amnestische Aphasie. Klinisches Bild und Überlegungen zur neurolinguistischen Struktur. J Neurol 207: 1, 1974.
10. Poeck, K., Huber, W., Kerschensteiner, M., Stachowiak, F.-J. & Weniger, D.: Therapie der Aphasien. Nervenarzt 48: 119, 1977.
11. Sies, L.: Aphasia Theory and Therapy: Selected lectures and papers of Hildred Schuell. University Park Press, Baltimore, 1974.
12. Stachowiak, F.-J., Huber, W., Kerschensteiner, M., Poeck, K., Weniger, D.: Die globale Aphasie. Klinisches Bild und Überlegungen zur neurolinguistischen Struktur. J Neurol 214: 75, 1977.
13. Wiegel-Crump, C.: Agrammatism and aphasia. In: Y. Lebrun & R. Hoops (eds.), Recovery in Aphasics, pp. 243–253. Swets & Zeitlinger, Amsterdam, 1976.
14. Wiegel-Crump, C. & Koenigsknecht, R.: Tapping the lexical store of the adult aphasic: Analysis of the improvement made in word retrieval skills. Cortex 9: 410, 1973.

The Token Test and the Reporter's Test: A measure of verbal input and a measure of verbal output

ENNIO DE RENZI

The Token Test

The first part of this paper presents normative data of a short version of the Token Test, a test developed in 1962 by De Renzi and Vignolo (1) to detect receptive disturbances in aphasics.

The original version of the Token Test consisted of 61 items, 10 with two words (touch the red circle), 10 with three words (touch the small white circle), 10 with four words (touch the yellow circle and the red rectangle), 10 with six words (touch the large yellow rectangle and the small green rectangle) and 21 with more complex instructions. This 61 item-version has been deemed too long by several investigators, and shorter versions have been proposed, either by reducing the length of each part, or by eliminating one or more parts. Spellacy and Spreen (2) have provided evidence that a 16-item version of the test is approximately as effective as the original presentation in separating aphasic from non-aphasic brain-damaged patients. Capitalizing on this experience we have developed a 36-item version of the test. The first 7 items are new and involve commands simpler than any of those used in the original version, since they require understanding only one word. This part has been introduced with the aim of permitting a more graded evaluation of the patient's comprehension deficit and avoiding the "floor effect" produced by the test when it is given to severe aphasics. Other minor modifications are the substitution of rectangles by squares, which are more familiar to patients, and of the blue tokens by black ones, as it has been shown that brain-damaged patients may experience some difficulty in distinguishing blue from green (3). Fig. 1 shows the arrangement of the tokens. The commands are as follows:

Part 1 (*All 20 tokens are presented*)

1. Touch a circle
2. Touch a square
3. Touch a red token
4. Touch a yellow one
5. Touch a white one
6. Touch a green one
7. Touch a black one

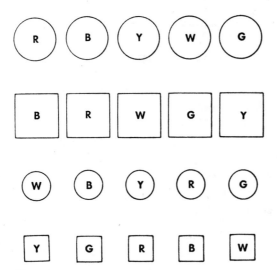

Fig. 1. Arrangement of tokens.

Part 2 (*Large tokens only are presented*)

8. Touch the yellow square
9. Touch the black circle
10. Touch the green circle
11. Touch the white square

Part 3. (*All 20 tokens are presented*)

12. Touch the small white circle
13. Touch the large yellow square
14. Touch the large green square
15. Touch the small black circle

Part 4. (*Large tokens only are presented*)

16. Touch the red circle and the green square
17. Touch the yellow square and the black square
18. Touch the white square and the green circle
19. Touch the white circle and the red circle

Part 5. (*All 20 tokens are presented*)

20. Touch the large white circle and the small green square
21. Touch the small black circle and the large yellow square
22. Touch the large green square and the large red square
23. Touch the large white square and the small green circle

Part 6. (*Large tokens only are presented*)

24. Put the red circle on the green square
25. Touch the black circle with the red square

26. Touch the black circle and the red square
27. Touch the black circle or the red square
28. Put the green square away from the yellow square
29. If there is a blue circle, touch the red square.
    (N.B. There is no blue circle)
30. Put the green square near the red circle
31. Touch the squares, slowly, and the circles, quickly
32. Put the red circle between the yellow square and the green square
33. Except for the green one, touch the circles
34. Touch the red circle—no!—the white square
35. Instead of the white square, touch the yellow circle
36. Together with the yellow circle, touch the black circle

The commands of part 1 to 5 may be repeated once, if wrongly performed. One point is credited for a correct performance at the first presentation; 0.5 points for a correct performance at the second presentation. No repetition of the command is permitted for part 6. The total score can range from 0 to 36.

Results

Control patients

The test was given to 215 control patients. The influence of age and years of schooling on performance was assessed by computing the regression coefficients of the test scores on these factors. Age had a negligible regression coefficient of -0.03, e.g. a 70-year-old subject would be expected to score only 1.50 points less than a 20-year-old subject. The regression coefficient (0.30) for years of schooling was more substantial. This indicates that a subject with 17 years of schooling would be expected to score 4.20 points more than a subject with 3 years of schooling. Only years of schooling were, therefore, taken into account in establishing the cutting score which discriminates normal from pathological performances. Normal subjects were divided into 4 groups: 3–5 yrs of schooling, 6–8 yrs of schooling, 9–12 yrs of schooling and more than 12 yrs of schooling (Table I). For each group the mean and standard deviation were computed. The cut off score was set at the level of performance corresponding to the mean minus 2 S.D. Only 2.5% of the normal population would be expected to fall below this score. The cutting score was 27 for the group with 3–5 yrs of schooling, 29 for the group with 6–8 yrs of schooling, 30 for the group with 9–12 yrs of schooling and 32 for the group with more than 12 yrs of schooling.

Right and left non-aphasic brain-damaged patients

The test was given to 130 patients with right hemisphere damage. Nineteen patients (15%) fell below the cut off score of the corresponding control

Table I. *Distribution of the control patients' scores*

Score	3–5 yrs schooling (N=100)	6–8 yrs schooling (N=45)	9–12 yrs schooling (N=37)	12 yrs schooling (N=33)
36	2	3	2	14
35	7	7	12	9
34	20	7	7	9
33	16	9	8	—
32	17	8	4	—
31	15	5	1	—
30	12	4	2	—
29	3	—	1	1
28	1	1		
27	2	1		
26	2			
25	—			
24	1			
23	—			
22	1			
21	1			
$\bar{X}$	31.82	32.76	33.57	34.97
S.D.	2.66	2.05	1.69	1.36

groups, usually no more than 1–5 points (Table II). The only patients who scored more poorly were those with clinical signs of unilateral visual neglect, a deficit which is likely to interfere with the exploration of a whole array of tokens. Fifty left brain-damaged patients, considered free from aphasia on the basis of clinical examination and a standard aphasia examination, were also given the test. Nine (18 %) fell below the cut off scores, usually no more than 5 points (Table III).

Aphasic patients

One hundred and six aphasic patients were examined. Their scores were extremely scattered, ranging from 0 to 35 points. The mean was 14.37, S.D. 8.90. Only 10 (9 %) had scores above or at the level of the cutoff scores and would be, therefore, considered non aphasic on the basis of their Token Test performance. This percentage may be compared with that of 40 %, found in the same patients when they were given a 10 sentence comprehension test, included in the standard aphasia examination and for which a 5 % cutoff score was also available. We adopted the aphasics' mean (14) as the score distinguishing global from Broca aphasics among the patients whose speech is not fluent and severe Wernicke from other Wernicke aphasics among patients whose speech is fluent. This classification is currently used in our department

Table II. *Distribution of the right brain-damaged patients' scores*

Score	3–5 yrs schooling (N=79)	6–8 yrs schooling (N=31)	9–12 yrs schooling (N=9)	12 yrs schooling (N=11)
36	1	3	1	4
35	10	7	1	1
34	7	4	1	3
33	7	7	2	1
32	13	2	2	
31	10	2	1	
30	7	2		
29	7	1		
28	3			
27	2	1		
26	1			2
25	3			
24	2	1°	1	
23	1			
22	2			
21		1°	1	
20	1°			
19	1°			
...				
15	1°			
$\bar{X}$	30.41	32.48	32.22	33.27
S.D.	4.13	3.44	3.46	2.74

and rests upon the rules set forth on the basis of the findings of the standard aphasia examination (4). Table IV shows the number of patients in these four categories who fall above and below the score of 14. The agreement between the two criteria of classification appears to be satisfactory.

The Reporter's Test

The ability of aphasic patients to comunicate verbally can be assessed with a number of tasks. Some of them require the recall of a given word in a typical stimulus-response condition: e.g. naming visually presented objects; answering with a name to a question; providing the opposite of a substantive, adjective or adverb, etc. These tasks are sensitive to anomia and easy to score but they do not permit evaluating the patient's capacity to produce words in connected sequences, and, consequently, the fluency of his speech. Fluency is better evaluated by engaging the patient in spontaneous conversation or providing him with a stimulus for a short narrative description. In our laboratory we requested the patient to describe (if a man) how he would shave himself, or

Table III. *Distribution of non-aphasic left brain-damaged patients' scores*

Score	3–5 yrs schooling (N=18)	6–8 yrs schooling (N=18)	9–12 yrs schooling (N=4)	12 yrs schooling (N=10)
36		1	1	
35		1	1	4
34	4		1	3
33	2	3		2
32		3		1
31	3	1		
30	1	4		
29	3	1	1	
28	1	2		
27		1		
26	1			
25				
24	1			
23				
22	1	1		
21				
20	1			
$\bar{X}$	29.56	30.61	33.50	34
S.D.	4.23	3.22	3.11	1.05

(if a woman) how she would cook spaghetti. Goodglass and Kaplan (5) present the patient with a picture situation with instructions to tell all about what he sees happening in the picture. While the verbal material derived from these procedures is suited for a qualitative evaluation, it presents problems of quantification and objective scoring. Even normal people differ remarkably from each other in their tendency to elaborate and to go into details when asked to speak on a topic, some of them being laconic, others prolix. Moreover, emotional problems or mood disturbances (not rare among brain-damaged patients) can produce inhibition and result in a poverty of spontaneous expression, which leaves the examiner uncertain about the linguistic competence of the subject.

Table IV. *Number of patients, belonging to the different aphasic categories, who score above or below the mean*

	Global	Broca	Severe Wernicke	Mild to moderate Wernicke
⩾14	1	26	4	23
<14	22	4	19	7

An ideal test should provide objective criteria to determine how many and which words the subject must produce to answer a question adequately. We investigated the possibility of meeting these requirements with a new test we propose to call "The Reporter's Test". It asks the patient to act as a reporter of the actions carried out by the examiner, as if he had to describe what is happening to a third person who cannot see. The examiner's performance corresponds to the Token Test commands and utilizes the material of the Token Test.

Subjects

Forty subjects admitted for disease not involving the central nervous system made up the control group. Their mean age was 46.15 years, their mean years of schooling was 7.53 years.

Aphasics were considered eligible to participate in this investigation only if their speech output was not severely impaired. There were 24 such patients. Their mean age was 56.71, their mean years of schooling was 5.83.

Procedure

The Token Test was always administered first, in order to acquaint the subject with the kind of material and commands he was subsequently to describe. The 20 tokens were laid down on the table in the same arrangement used in the receptive version of the test (Fig. 1). The following instructions were given to control patients:

"Now, I am going to do some things with these tokens. Imagine that a person is sitting beside you, but is prevented from seeing what I do by a curtain (the examiner shields the tokens with a cardboard vertically held). Your task is to describe what I am doing as carefully as possible, so that this person would be able to do exactly what I do on another set of tokens. As you see, there are circles and squares, some are large and some small, some are yellow, others red, black, green and white. Therefore, if I touch this token (the E points to the black small square), you cannot simply call it a square or the black square but you have to say "the small black square". A few examples are given and the subject's report is corrected if wrong.

The procedure followed with aphasics was different. A second examiner sat besides the patient with an array of tokens in front of him; a carboard prevented him from viewing the various performances of the first examiner, although he actually knew them. The patient was told that he had to describe what the first examiner did with the tokens as precisely as possible, because the second examiner would try to repeat the performance on his own array of tokens, on the basis of the information given by the patient. Whenever the description was incomplete or ambiguous, the second examiner (who in fact knew from a concealed sheet which was the right command) deliberately chose the wrong alternative. The second examiner's behavior provided, therefore, a feedback to the patient on the correctness of his report.

The test

The test is made up of five parts, some requiring all the twenty tokens (arranged as in Fig. 1) and some only the large tokens. The performances carried out in the first four parts correspond to the commands given in part 2–3–4–5 of the Token Test. The examiner touches one or two tokens, which requires the patient to construct a sentence with a simple syntactic structure: verb (always the same: "touch") and object, this last varying from one to two substantives and from one to four adjectives. Part five has 10 items, some derived from part six of the Token Test and some new. It was appreciated that some commands of part six of the Token Test would have changed their linguistic formulation, when performed by the examiner. For example, the command "Touch the black circle or the red square" would result in the patient's report "Touch the black circle" or "Touch the red square" according to the examiner's choice. Consequently, only 7 original items were retained and 3 new items were added. The sentences originated by the corresponding performances involve, in addition to the substantives and adjectives designating the tokens, two verbs ("touch" or "put"), prepositions and adverbs.

The items of part 5 are reported with the formulation the patient is expected to give.

Part 5. (*Large tokens only*)

17. Put the red circle on the green square
18. Put the circles on the squares of the corresponding color
19. Put the green square away from the yellow square
20. Put the green square near the red circle
21. Touch the squares slowly and the circles quickly
22. Put the red circle among the yellow and green square
23. Touch all the circles, except the green one
24. Put the yellow square under the black circle
25. Put all the circles into the box
26. Put the squares one on the other

Scoring

If the patient's description is erroneous or incomplete, the performance is repeated. One point is credited for a correct description given after the first performance, 0.5 point if the description is initially wrong, but is corrected after the second performance.

Scoring the responses of the first four parts of the test did not raise any problem, except for the fact that some patients, both controls and aphasics, forgot to mention the verb "touch" after the first items. This behavior was not penalized.

The patient's description of some items of part five did not always correspond to the originally conceived formulation. On the ground of the control subjects' performance, the following reports, although heterodox, have been considered acceptable, and they may assist as guidelines for other idiosyncratic responses.

Item 17: none.
Item 18: enumeration of the ten tokens, i.e.: put the red circle on the red square, the green circle on the green square etc.
Item 19: whenever the subject says "move, put away, take away etc. the green square" without mentioning the yellow square.
Item 20: "besides" instead of "near".
Item 21: enumeration of each of the ten tokens, provided it is specified that the squares must be touched slowly, and the circle quickly.
Item 22: none.
Item 23: enumeration of the four circles that must be touched.
Item 24: "put the yellow square in the place of the black circle and the black circle on the yellow square". Simply saying "put the black circle on the yellow square" would be wrong, because it implies that the circle and not the square must be moved.
Item 25: none.
Item 26: enumeration of the five squares, or "pick up the squares and make a pile of them". It must be clear that the squares must be piled up and not simply heaped.

Results

Controls

The regression of the scores on age and educational level was computed. The regression coefficient for age was 0.016 and fell far short of being significant; that for years of schooling was —0.185 and was significant ($p < 0.025$). To partial out the influence of educational level the scores have been corrected according to the following formula: observed score $+1.39 - (0.18 \times \text{years of schooling})$.

The adjusted scores of control patients had a mean of 23.36, S.D. 1.65. In order to establish a cut off score discriminating normal from pathological performances, the 98%, 95% and 90% confidence intervals of the control scores were computed: the percentage of the normal population that would be expected to fall below them is 1%, 2.5% and 5%, respectively. This statement entails a risk of error <5%. The 1% cut off score is 18, the 2.5% cut off score is 18.75, the 5% cut off score is 19.39. One control patient was found to score lower than 19.39, the 5% cut off score, none lower than the 2.5% and 1% cut off scores.

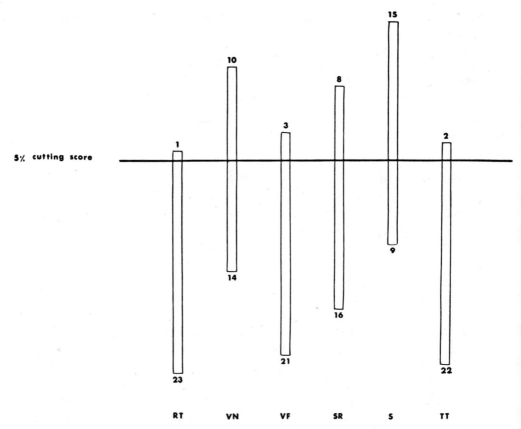

Fig. 2. Distribution of aphasic patients above and below the 5% cutting score on the Reporter's Test and on other verbal tests. *RT*, Reporter's Test; *VN*, visual naming; *VF*, verbal fluency; *SR*, sentence repetition; *S*, story; *TT*, Token Test.

Aphasics

The aphasics' scores were corrected for the effect of years of schooling with the above-mentioned formula. Their corrected mean was 10.56 (S.D. 6.27). One aphasic had a score of 19.73, which is higher than the 5% cutoff score. A second aphasic had a score of 18.67, which is higher than the 1% cut off score. All other aphasic patients performed at a lower level. Thus, the 5% cutting score misclassified 2 patients (1 control and 1 aphasic patient) out of 64 (3.12%), while the 1% cutoff score classified all controls correctly and misclassified 1 aphasic patient (1.56%). The diagnostic power of the Reporter's Test was compared to that of other expressive speech tests which had been given to the aphasic patients. They were: (1) a 20-item visual naming test, (2) an oral fluency test: saying all the words beginning with three given letters (P, F, L), allowing one minute for each letter, (3) a 21 item sentence repetition test, (4) a tell-a-story test. For each of these tests a 5% cutoff score, computed on a sample of 150 control patients, was available. Fig. 2 shows the distribution

Table V. *Correlation coefficients between the Reporter's Test and other tests in aphasic patients*

Visual naming	Fluency	Sentence repetition	Story	Token Test
.41*	.17	.32	.49*	.66***

* $p<0.05$.   *** $p<0.001$.

of the 24 aphasic patients above and below the 5% cutoff score on the Reporter's Test, the other expressive tests and the Token Test.

The percentage of aphasics not identified as such was 4% for the Reporter's Test, 42% for the visual naming test, 12% for the oral fluency test, 33% for the sentence repetition test, 62% for the tell-a-story test, and 8% for the Token Test. The only expressive test approaching the diagnostic power of the Reporter's Test was the oral fluency test, but this test is not specific for aphasia, as shown by previous research (6, 7, 8), where it has been found to be sensitive also to right brain damage and to damage involving left prefrontal areas.

Table V indicates the correlation coefficient between the Reporter's Test and the other tests in the aphasic sample.

In conclusion, these preliminary findings suggest that the Reporter's Test is an effective tool for diagnosing mild to moderate disorders of verbal expression, since it provides verbal material suited for both a qualitative and quantitative analysis. We are currently collecting data on the performances of right and left non-aphasic brain-damaged patients. We are also exploring the possibility of giving the test to aphasics without the presence of the second examiner, a condition which would greatly facilitate its utilization in routine practice. Preliminary data suggest that this change in procedure does not significantly affect the aphasics' performance.

Summary

The first part of this paper deals with the performance on a 36 item version of the Token Test of 215 control patients, 130 right brain-damaged patients, 50 left brain-damaged patients without clinical evidence of aphasia and 106 aphasic patients. Cutting scores discriminating a normal from an aphasic performance have been established for each of the four educational levels into which the subjects of this study were subdivided. Only 9.5% of the aphasics did not show comprehension deficit on the Token Test on the basis of these cutting scores. This percentage may be compared with the 40% of patients who scored in the normal range when the same aphasic sample was given a 10 sentence comprehension test. Right brain-damaged patients scored poorly only when suffering from severe visual neglect.

The second part of the paper presents preliminary data obtained with a new test, designed to evaluate expressive impairment in aphasia. It is derived from the Token Test and is named the Reporter Test, because it requires the patient to act as a reporter of the performances carried out by the examiner with the tokens. The patient's task is to verbally describe the performance with sufficient precision to permit a second examiner, who is prevented from seeing the first, to reproduce the same actions on a comparable array of tokens.

Forty control patients and 25 aphasic patients, selected on the basis of a mild to moderate expressive disorder, have been given the test. All but one aphasic scored lower than the worst performing control. This result compares favourably with those obtained on other speech tests (visual naming, verbal controlled associations, sentence repetition, tell-a-story), on all of which the percentage of aphasics that scored within the normal range was greater.

References

1. De Renzi, E. & Vignolo, L. A.: The Token Test: a sensitive test to detect receptive disturbances in aphasics. Brain 85: 665, 1962.
2. Spellacy, F. J. & Spreen, O.: A short form of the Token Test. Cortex 5: 390, 1969.
3. Scotti, G. & Spinnler, H.: Colour imperception in unilateral hemisphere-damaged patients. J Neurol Neuros Psychiat 33: 22, 1970.
4. Faglioni, P., Spinnler, H. & Vignolo, L. A.: Contrasting behavior of right and left hemisphere-damaged patients on a discriminative and a semantic task of auditory recognition. Cortex 5: 366, 1969.
5. Goodglass, H. & Kaplan, E.: The Assessment of Aphasia and Related Disorders. Lea and Febiger, Philadelphia, 1972.
6. Benton, A. L.: Differential behavioral effects in frontal lobe disease. Neuropsychologia 6: 53, 1968.
7. Boller, F.: Latent aphasia: right and left "non aphasic' brain-damaged patients compared. Cortex 4: 324, 1968.
8. Ramier, A. M. & Hécaen, H.: Rôle respectif des atteintes frontales et de la latéralisation lésionelle dans les deficits de "la fluence verbale". Rev Neurol 123: 17, 1970.

A therapy program for impairment of the use of the *kana*-syllabary of Japanese aphasic patients

SUMIKO SASANUMA

1. *Introduction*

Linguistic impairments induced by aphasia may reflect certain features which are uniquely related to the native language of the patient, as well as characteristics that are more or less universally recognized in different languages of the world. Certain aspects of reading and writing impairments exhibited by Japanese patients constitute an example of the former.

The Japanese orthography is unique in that two types of nonalphabetic symbols, *kana*[1] (phonetic symbols for syllables or morae[2]) and *kanji* (or Chinese characters, which are essentially non-phonetic, logographic symbols representing lexical morphemes), are used in combination, and this dual nature of the orthography sometimes creates certain types of dissociations between the processing of *kana* versus *kanji* characters among brain damaged patients. That is to say, in these patients one of the two types of writing systems can be impaired disproportionately to that of the other, resulting in the selective impairment of *kana* processing on the one hand, or the selective impairment of *kanji* processing on the other. Between these two extremes the more or

---

[1] There are two sets of 68 *kana* characters, *hiragana* and *katakana*, which are completely equivalent to one another (somewhat as the upper and lower case letters of an alphabet are equivalent, although the *katakana* set is used primarily for representing loanwords and in other contexts where one might use italics). Children learn to handle these two sets of *kana* characters first (usually by the end of the first grade in primary school) and then start learning *kanji* characters, which are used in writing primarily lexical morphemes. Due to the large number of *kanji* characters it is not unusual that even a highly educated person sometimes finds himself unable to recall some low-frequency *kanji* words, and represents them in *kana* instead. The converse situation never happens, however, i.e., because of the one-to-one correspondence existing between *kana* characters and morae, a normal literate person will have no difficulty in transcribing any Japanese words in *kana* as long as he knows the phonetic forms of the words.

[2] Japanese utterances are traditionally analyzed as consisting of morae, each mora consisting of either consonant plus vowel, vowel alone, mora nasal or mora obstruent, so that *hoo*, *hon*, and *ʔippon* are respectively 2, 2 and 4 morae (ho-o, ho-n, ʔi-p-po-n). Some of the reasons why the notion of mora is used in describing standard Japanese are: (1) the mora functions as the unit of length in the language, so that the length of a phrase is roughly proportional to the number of morae it contains; (2) the acoustic realization of accent in Japanese can only be described by stating which morae are high or low pitched; and (3) Japanese has phonological rules which depend on the number of morae rather than syllables.

less non-selective impairment of both *kana* and *kanji* can be observed as well (7).

This paper will attempt to describe a therapy program specifically developed for patients with selective impairment of *kana* processing, and will discuss some of the implications of the outcome of this approach.

2. *Nature of the selective impairment of* kana *processing and the theoretical background for the* kana *therapy program*

The selective impairment of *kana* processing does not emerge as an isolated disorder, but is typically embedded in a cluster of symptoms known as Broca's aphasia. Since one of the characteristics of these patients is that their speech is nonfluent and effortful with marked disturbance of phoneme production, in addition to the fact that they have the *kana* problem, we proposed a hypothesis that the impairment of the phonological component of the language may constitute a common source of these disabilities (5). In an attempt to pursue this issue further, an analysis was made of the error data obtained from a group of patients on the task of writing a set of words in *kana* as well as in *kanji*. The results indicated that there was an essential difference in the nature of errors between the two types of transcriptions. In *kana* the majority of errors were those which can best be explained in terms of some underlying 'phonological confusions' involving syllables, phonemes or distinctive features, while on the *kanji* task 'graphical confusions' constituted the most frequent type of errors (6).

Table I illustrates some examples of *kana* errors. As can be seen in Table I, the predominant errors are those where the target *kana* characters are replaced by other *kana* characters of similar phonemic values, i.e., one or two features apart. Transpositions (or metatheses) of adjacent or nonadjacent syllables, phonemes, or distinctive features constitute another type. Moreover, the majority of these phonological errors tend to be related to their phonological contexts (e.g., an assimilative influence of neighboring sounds). In other words, the disintegration of *kana* processing takes place not at random, but in a highly orderly fashion which is predictable from the phonological principles of the language. And this is exactly the kind of orderliness one would expect to find in the 'articulation' errors or phonemic errors of these patients in their oral language in general (1, 2, 8). These findings taken together seem to provide further evidence in support of the hypothesis of the phonological basis of *kana* impairment.

It is this hypothesis that we have drawn upon as a theoretical framework for developing the *kana* retraining program. According to this framework, the therapeutic intervention is focused directly on the phonological aspect of the language, and not just on the reading and writing of *kana* characters in the conventional sense. Whatever efficacy that is expected of this therapy,

Table I. *An analysis of* kana *errors exhibited by Broca's aphasics in terms of distinctive features*

Target Words	Responses	Analyses
	て い と te	$k \to t/\_\_\_t$ (p)[*]
け い と	け い こ 　　ko	$t \to k/k\_\_\_$ (p)
ke i to		
(yarn)	て い こ te　ko	$k \to t/\_\_\_t$ $t \to k/k\_\_\_$　(p)
	と ど も to	$k \to t/\_\_\_d$ (p)
こ ど も	こ の も 　no	$d \to n/\_\_\_m$ (p)
ko do mo		
(child)	こ の ぼ 　no bo	$d \to n/\_\_\_m$ $m \to b/d\_\_\_$　(n)[**]
	け ぶ く ろ ke	$t \to k/\_\_\_k$ (p)
て ぶ く ろ	て ぷ く ろ 　pu	$b \to p/t\_\_k$ (v)[***]
te bu ku ro		
(gloves)	て く ぶ ろ 　ku bu	$b \to k/\_\_\_k$ $k \to b/b\_\_\_$　(v,p)
	テ ク タ イ te	$n \to t/\_\_\_t$ (n,v)
ネ ク タ イ	テ ク ナ イ te　na	$n \to t/\_\_\_t$ $t \to n/n\_\_\_$　(n,v)
ne ku ta i		
(necktie)		
	ぜ い ろ う こ ze　ro	$r \to z/\_\_\_z$ $z \to r/r\_\_\_$　(m)[****]
れ い ぞ う こ		
re i zo o ko	れ い ご う こ 　　go	$z \to g/\_\_\_k$ (p,m)
(refrigerator)		

---

[*]	(p): place	[***]	(v): voicing
[**]	(n): nasality	[****]	(m): manner

therefore, should be two-fold, i.e., it should bring about the improvement not only of *kana* processing but also of phoneme production and reception as well.

3. *Retraining Procedures*

3.1. Evaluation of *kana* impairment: Phonemic Segmentation Test

One of the diagnostic tests that we have developed for use in identifying candidates for this *kana* therapy program is called the Phonemic Segmentation Test (4). With this test we seek to assess the patient's ability at analyzing speech into its component morae (or syllables) as well as singling out a given mora from its surrounding context. It consists of two parts. In part I, the patient is given a spoken list of 3-mora words and is asked whether he hears the /ka/ mora in each word (Table II *a*).

In part II he is given only those words which contain a /ka/ mora either in the initial, the middle, or the final position of the words, and asked to point to one of the three circles, shown in Table II *b*, where he thinks the /ka/ is located (Table II *b*).

The data accumulated thus far indicate that the scores on this test are distributed over a continuum out of which at least two groups of patients can be identified on the basis of their level of performance on this test, namely, a poor performance group and a good performance group. The majority of the patients falling into the poor performance group are those with Broca's aphasia, who invariably show severe impairment of 'articulation' or phoneme production, and of *kana* processing. In other words, those who have a selective impairment of *kana* processing tend to exhibit, at the same time, a marked difficulty of 'articulation' as well as in analyzing speech into its component sound units, indicating a close association between these abilities.

The majority of patients in the good performance group, on the other hand, are those who belong to some subgroup of fluent aphasia, such as anomic or conduction aphasias or a mild form of Wernicke's aphasia, and they have a nonselective mild to moderate impairment of both *kana* and *kanji* processing. Their level of performance on the Phonemic Segmentation Test tends to be significantly better than that of the poor performance group, in spite of the fact that their *kana* processing impairment might not necessarily be very mild in the beginning. Fig. 1 shows this relationship. The ordinate represents the percentage of correct responses on the task of writing individual *kana* characters to dictation, while the abscissa represents the percentage of correct responses on the Phonemic Segmentation Test. As can be seen, a fairly strong positive correlation is demonstrated between the two tasks ($r = 0.79$).

Follow-up data obtained with a limited number of patients thus far indicate that the performance on the Phonemic Segmentation Test (PST) has a high

Table II. *Phonemic Segmentation Test: Parts I and II*

PART I

DO YOU HEAR A /ka/ SOUND?

Three-mora words	Response Yes	No
hi ka ri	___	___
a hi ru	___	___
mo na ka	___	___
ka ta na	___	___
ba na na	___	___
su ru me	___	___
.	.	.
.	.	.
.	.	.
.	.	.

PART II

WHERE IS THE /ka/ SOUND?

Three-mora words	Response		
i ka da	O	O	O
ka ga mi	O	O	O
hi ka ri	O	O	O
ga i ka	O	O	O
mo na ka	O	O	O
ka ta na	O	O	O
.		.	
.		.	
.		.	
.		.	
.		.	

prognostic value for *kana* impairment. That is to say, the prognosis for those patients whose PST scores fall below 70% should be guarded, in the sense that unless they are exposed to a special kind of retraining program the level of recovery of *kana* processing that can be attained by them is apt to stay rather low, just barely functional at best. In other words, these are the patients who make the best candidates for our kana therapy.

In contrast, the prognosis for those patients who demonstrate good performance (above 70%) on the PST tends to be quite promising even without

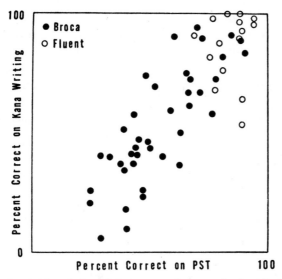

Fig. 1. The relationship between performance level on the Phonemic Segmentation Test and on the task of writing individual *kana* characters to dictation for aphasic patients.

being enrolled in a special program, and most of them are able to attain a functional level of *kana* processing in a relatively short period of time (say, 3–4 months).

3.2. Kana therapy program

As has just been pointed out, the PST data tell us that there are at least two groups of aphasic patients whose recovery courses for *kana* impairment are predicted to be clearly different and thus call for different therapeutic procedures. The patients in the poor PST performance group have to go through a rather laborious course of intensive retraining, consisting of analytic step-by-step procedures; while in the case of the majority of patients in the good performance group, it usually suffices to work with them in the framework of a general stimulation approach.

In this section, I am going to describe in some detail our analytic approach (3), which was specifically designed for patients who show poor performance on the PST as well as on the *kana* test. The program consists of five steps of graded difficulty, all of which are directed to the goal of improving the patient's ability in three major areas: (1) to analyze speech into its component sound-units (i.e., morae or syllables); (2) to match them with corresponding components of written speech (i.e., *kana* characters); and conversely (3) to synthesize these component-units into meaningful, integral wholes, such as words.

In step 1, we select a few key words in *kana* and familiarize the patient with them thoroughly, so that he can recognize them, can repeat, read and write them freely and with ease. In step 2, the patient is trained to become aware of the fact that each word is made up of component morae and to be able to analyze each word into these morae. For this purpose, we use various activities to make the patient identify each mora in a word and single it out from its context or sound sequence. These activities include tapping the desk, drawing a circle, or placing a marble, for each mora of the word spoken by the therapist. In step, 3, the patient is introduced to the one-to-one correspondence that exists between a mora and a *kana* character. In order to help him grasp this mora-grapheme relationship and strengthen the association between the two, various activities are used again, such as locating a *kana* symbol spoken by the therapist in a word or on a display of a few randomized *kana* symbols, etc. Step 4 is intended for synthesizing isolated morae into a meaningful sequences such as a word. The patient is asked to construct a word with a set of *kana* symbols presented randomly, or he is asked to read a word written in *kana*, not as a string of separate morae as he often does, but as an integral, meaningful whole. Throughout these steps we make full use of the key words, starting with them at every step and then gradually expanding this core, to incorporate other, more difficult, words. Step 5 is a graded application of those skills mastered in the previous steps to practical situations, such as reading and writing phrases, simple sentences and paragraphs in a variety of life situations.

As I mentioned earlier, this is a slow and laborious process, but we have seen many patients who could achieve a sizeable improvement in both *kana* processing and phonemic production/reception abilities only through these step-by-step analytic procedures.

3.3. A case report

In order to illustrate the actual recovery course of the patients enrolled in this program, a brief presentation will be made of a case of Broca's aphasia (3). This patient was a 37 year old housewife whose aphasia was of vascular etiology. On the linguistic evaluation made 3 months post onset, she showed a typical profile of Broca's aphasia accompanied by severe impairment of *kana* processing (Fig. 2), and was assigned to our *kana* therapy program on a 1-hour, 3 session/week basis.

Fig. 3 shows the month-by-month improvement in her performance levels on three tasks (repetition of syllables, reading individual *kana* characters aloud, and writing individual *kana* characters to dictation, all of which involve some kind of phonological processing). There are two important observations that can be made from this figure.

In the first place, it will be seen that the performance levels of the patient on all the three tasks improved parallel to each other throughout the training period. This is exactly what was predicted from the nature of the program, i.e., since the program is intended to work directly upon the phonological system, it should bring about an improvement not only in *kana* processing, but also in phoneme production/reception.

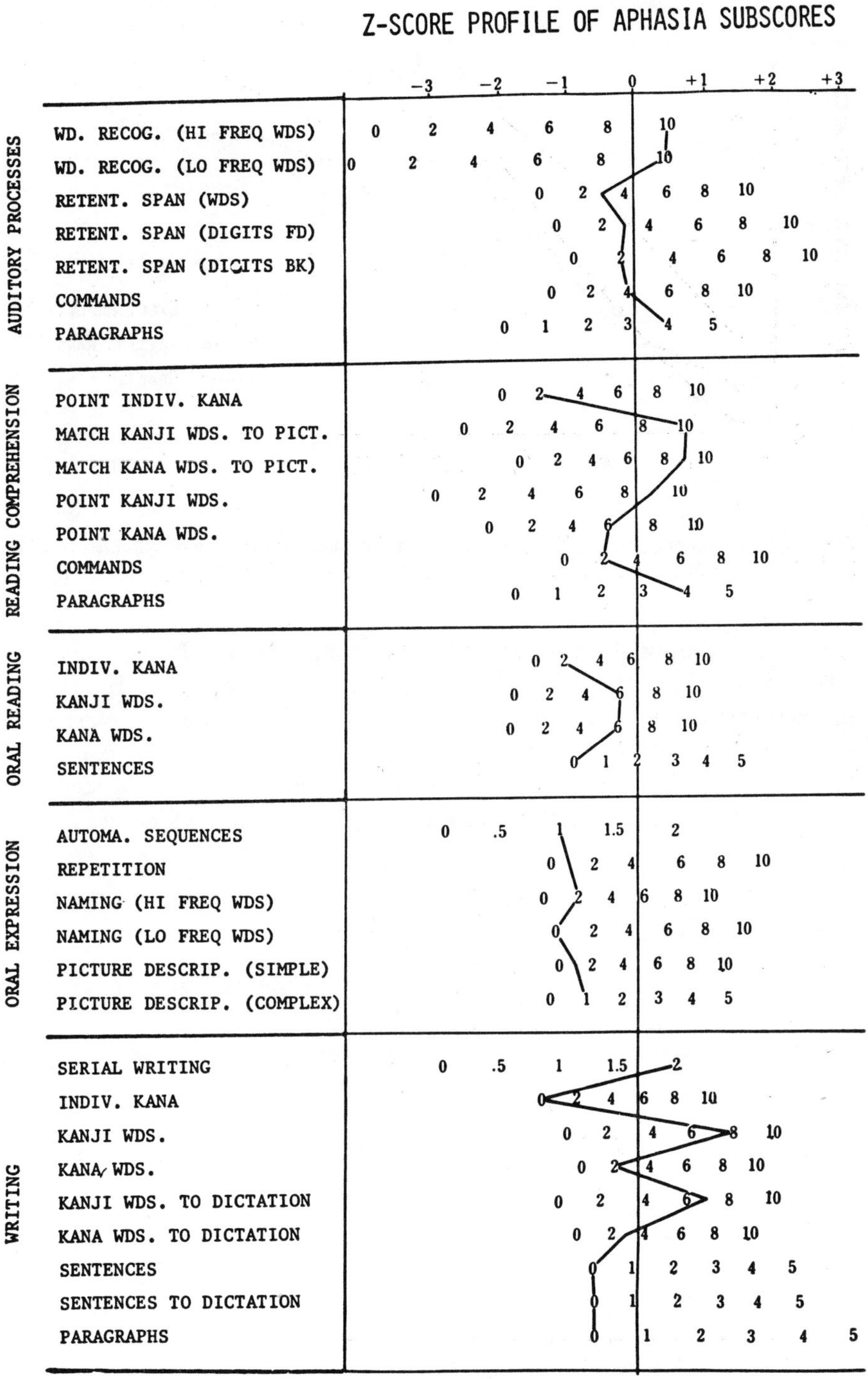

Fig. 2. Z-score profile of a Broca's aphasic (3 months post onset).

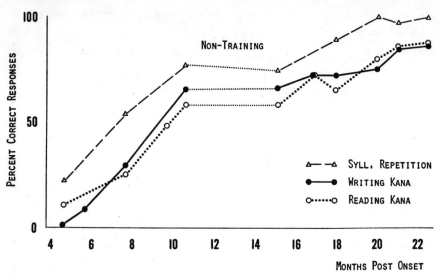

Fig. 3. The recovery course of a Broca's aphasic on three tasks: repetition of syllables, reading individual *kana* characters aloud, and writing individual *kana* characters to dictation (3).

Secondly, during the two and one-half month period of temporary discontinuation of the therapy (indicated by the dotted lines in the Fig. 3) the improvement came to a complete stop for all three tasks, while performance on other types of tasks such as 'naming' and 'describing pictures' continued to improve during the same period of non-training. This finding seems to indicate that there is a certain critical period in the recovery course during

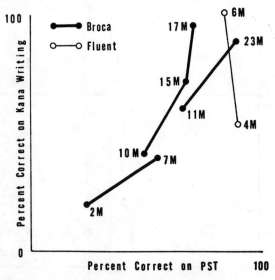

Fig. 4. The relationship between performance level on the Phonemic Segmentation Test and on the task of writing individual *kana* characters to dictation during the recovery course for three Broca's aphasics and one fluent aphasic.

which a training program of this sort is indispensable for the improvement of *kana* processing in severely impaired patients.

Fig. 4 shows the recovery course of a few additional patients with a selective impairment of *kana* processing. Again, the ordinate represents the *kana* writing ability and the abscissa the phonemic segmentation ability. As can be seen, in all the Broca's cases the improvement proceeds along a diagonal line, indicating a close relationship between the two abilities.

4. *Concluding remarks*

I have presented a hypothesis-oriented therapy program specifically designed for the selective impairment of *kana* processing and aimed at working directly upon the phonological system of the patient. The results of the application of this program to a group of patients thus far seem to provide further evidence in support of the validity of the theoretical framework on which the program was developed, i.e., the impairment of phonological processing constitutes an important underlying mechanism in disorders of *kana* processing as well as in disorders of phoneme production and reception.

The implications derived from these findings seem to be two-fold, highlighting the reciprocal merits of a hypothesis-testing approach in aphasia therapy. That is to say, by formulating an adequate hypothesis about the neuropsychological mechanisms underlying the symptom(s), one has a better chance of arriving at a more efficient therapeutic approach on the one hand, and through implementation of this approach in actual therapy one can test the validity or goodness of the hypothesis on the other. If the hypothesis is confirmed, we are closer to the understanding of the neuropsychological mechanisms of the impairment in question and obtaining further insight into the normal organization of language as well.

References

1. Blumstein, S.: Some phonological implications of aphasic speech. In: H. Goodglass and S. Blumstein (eds.), Psycholinguistics and Aphasia, pp. 123. Johns Hopkins University Press, Baltimore, 1973.
2. Blumstein, S. E.: A Phonological Investigation of Aphasic Speech. Mouton & Co., The Hague, 1973.
3. Monoi, H.: A *kana* training program for a patient with Broca's aphasia: a case report. Communication Disorder Research 5: 105, 1976. (In Japanese.)
4. Monoi, H. & Sasanuma, S.: Phonemic segmentation and *kana* processing in aphasic patients. Japan Journal of Logopedics and Phoniatrics 16: 169, 1975. (In Japanese.)
5. Sasanuma, S. & Fujimura, O.: Selective impairment of phonetic and non-phonetic transcription of words in Japanese aphasic patients: kana vs. kanji in visual recognition and writing. Cortex 7: 1, 1971.

6. Sasanuma, S. & Fujimura, O.: An analysis of writing errors in Japanese aphasic patients: kanji versus kana words. Cortex 8: 265, 1972.
7. Sasanuma, S.: Kana and kanji processing in Japanese aphasics. Brain and Language 2: 369, 1975.
8. Trost, J. & Canter, G. J.: Apraxia of speech in patients with Broca's aphasia: a study of phoneme production accuracy and error patterns. Brain and Language 1: 63, 1974.

Evaluation, outcome and treatment of aphasia in patients with severe head injuries

INGER VIBEKE THOMSEN

The question of reeducation of aphasics is a controversial one. Some believe that recovery, if any, is a spontaneous process in which retraining has no or minimal effect. Others, as Weisenburg and McBride (10) and Butfield and Zangwill (2), have published studies indicating that reeducation of language may influence the rate and extent of improvement. Vignolo (13), who was the first to include an objective assessment of an untreated group of aphasics, came to the same conclusion when retraining was given for at least six months.

The prognosis in traumatic aphasia is considered better than that of cerebrovascular disease. However, aphasics with severe head trauma present a variety of neuropsychological dysfunctions among which especially impairment of memory and learning may interfere with rehabilitation.

The purpose of the present investigation has been to evaluate and describe the outcome of aphasia in severely head injured patients, who received long-term reeducation, to discuss the indication hereof and the type of training.

Material and methods

In a series of 50 patients with severe head injuries previously described (6), 27 had symptoms of aphasia when seen for the first time on an average of four months after the trauma. Nearly all were victims of road accidents and the majority were men between 15 and 25 years. All but one patient was unconscious at the scene of accident and on admission to hospital and remained so for days or weeks. Only one aphasic had a P.T.A. of less than one month. 12 aphasics had closed head trauma and 15 had focal lesions, verified by operation. Half the patients with closed head trauma had permanent slow waves over the left temporal lobe or over both temporal lobes. Among the 15 patients with verified focal lesions, five had open brain injuries, eight had extracerebral hematoma, and two had intracerebral hemorrhage. It is of course reasonable to assume that also this group of patients had diffuse neuronal damage. As to the sites of the main lesions, there was a clear preponderance of lesions involving the left temporal lobe.

Testing of aphasia was not possible at the first examination when lack of spontaneity, severe bradyphrenia and regression were common features. The primary results were therefore based on observation for some weeks. The majority of aphasics were treated by the author for months or years, in several cases every second day. The general verbal stimulation approach was initially used to establish contact and to elicit response. Meaningful language units of common everyday words were presented orally in situations which were supposed to be familiar to the patient. If there was any reading ability, auditory and written stimuli were given simultaneously. The main stress was laid on afferent reactions, and speech was considered less important at the early stage. In patients with no or minimal cooperation, singing or Body-Ego-Technique, beginning with imitation of body movements and attempts of identification, were used. The stimulation approach was considered most important and was continued in various forms of increasing complexity, according to the individual patient's need, throughout the rehabilitation period. When it became possible, retraining of reading took place. The main stress was, however, laid on oral communication. Among the materials applied, one type proved highly useful. Series of pictures, six in number, illustrating the evolution of different themes from everyday life, were used to stimulate afferent and efferent aspects of communication. The pictures were presented in random order and the patient was asked to arrange them correctly, to point to the picture the clinician referred to (oral and/or written stimuli), and to give a verbal description of the story. In aphasics with severe impairment of speech the clinician formulated sentences from the words or fragments of sentences the patient produced. The tape recorder was used, when the play-back did not create frustration.

The author worked in close contact with the staff at the hospitals. The problems of communication were discussed and attempts were made to stimulate functional communication in the wards and in the different departments of rehabilitation. Information and advice was of course also given to relatives.

A follow-up examination took place two and a half years on an average after the trauma. The patients were visited in their homes, where they and their relatives were asked questions about functional communication. The patients were readmitted to hospital and seen by a neurologist, a clinical psychologist, and by the author, who performed tests of aphasia and verbal learning.

Results

Disorders of language were initially severe in the majority of patients. The defects of language and speech present at the first examination and at the follow-up examination are shown in Table I.

It is seen in the table that impaired analysis of speech and reading, amnestic aphasia, verbal paraphasia, agraphia, and perseveration were present in nearly all at the first examination and that these symptoms remained the most

Table I. *Defects of language and speech at first examination an* examination in 27 patients

Defects	Patients (no.)	
	1st exam.	Follow-up
Impaired analysis of speech	21	12
Impaired analysis of reading	21	12
Amnestic aphasia	23	20
Verbal paraphasia	22	15
Literal paraphasia	10	5
Paragrammatism	8	8
Agrammatism	2	2
Agraphia	21	9
Dysarthria	6	6
Perseveration	21	21
No symptoms	0	5[a]

[a] In test of aphasia.

outstanding ones. It is also seen that five patients presented no aphasic symptoms in the test at the follow-up. One patient with a subdural hematoma in the left temporal lobe and signs of very severe brainstem damage had very severe dysarthria. The primary diagnosis had been difficult to make (8). The four other patients had closed head trauma. Their spontaneous speech and verbal learning revealed aphasic traits (7, 9).

At the follow-up examination all aphasics with closed head trauma but one had amnestic aphasia. The remaining patient had sensory aphasia. In patients with verified focal lesions, amnestic aphasia was found in the majority, a few had sensory aphasia, and one had motor aphasia. The latter patient had an open brain injury with frontotemporal laceration. She was the only one in whom no improvement of functional communication occurred.

The types of aphasia changed in many patients in the interval between the two examinations. Total aphasia, in two patients with verified focal lesions, had become sensory aphasia, and sensory aphasia had changed into amnestic aphasia. Five patients with focal lesions were severely aphasic at the follow up. They had extensive lesions in the left hemisphere or lesions involving the left temporoparietal or frontotemporal regions. The others with focal lesions had moderate or mild aphasia. Among aphasics with closed head trauma, only the patient with sensory aphasia remained severely aphasic. She had permanent 2–4 Hz waves in the left parietooccipital region.

According to information from patients and/or relatives nine aphasics had impaired comprehension of oral language. One patient had trouble in simple conversation with one person, the others had difficulty in understanding speech on the telephone, television, and conversation with more than one person. Half the patients had difficulties in expressing themselves, mostly on account amnestic aphasia. All patients had trouble reading or took no interest. Only one or two tried to read books and very few read anything but newspaper headlines.

Discussion

The aphasic patient with severe head trauma differs in behaviour from the patient with aphasia following cerebrovascular disease. While the latter frequently realizes his problems of communication at a rather early stage, the former often remains totally unaware for months. Awareness of neuropsychological deficits comes gradually and slowly and sometimes only partially, and this fact must of course be taken into consideration in rehabilitation.

In the present study the stimulation approach has formed an important part of reeducation. Much stress has been placed on auditory stimulation, as so often suggested by Schuell et al. (4). The way of addressing the patient and the voice have been considered important factors, especially in the earlier stages. The rate of speech must not be too fast and yet not artificially slow. It is doubtful whether speaking in a loud voice helps the patient, but the emotional qualities of the voice, the interest and activation deliberately expressed in the manner of speaking, may play a decisive part. Even in total aphasia the patient may show some reaction to emotional, hyperprosodic speech (8). Direct language therapy is not possible in the early phase; correction of speech is for instance meaningless as long as the patient is totally unaware of his defects. However, it is impossible to agree with Wepman (12), when he says that therapy should not begin until the patient himself indicates a need. Stimulation must be given to all aphasics as soon as possible and also to non-aphasics with severe lack of spontaneity. Early contacts with the patient may provide the clinician with valuable information. Treatment and observation form a synthesis and the long-term observation of patients with severe head injuries often reveals features in verbal and non-verbal behaviour that may pass unnoticed in the testing situation. The patient's reaction to treatment is of course also most important. Wepman (11) thus finds that the ability to be stimulated is a highly valuable prognostic parameter.

In the present study reeducation of oral language was considered the main thing. Retraining of functions that have been acquired later in life, such as reading, may have limited value in patients with severe brain damage. Some aphasics in the investigation had only a few errors in the test of silent reading, but their speed of reading was extremely slow. They had to reread again and again. The very low verbal retention span (9) certainly had an overall effect on language functions. Even aphasics with rather mild reduction of verbal retention span may lose interest in reading, because they cannot remember what they are reading (5). Premorbid level of education and premorbid interest in reading are of course also factors of great influence.

At the follow-up the majority of patients had amnestic aphasia. This type of aphasia is a common end-stage of evolution, whatever the ætiology, as described by Kertesz and McCabe (3), and this may particularly apply to patients with severe head trauma. As to the severity, the results in this long-term study indicate that only head injured patients with severe focal lesions in the so-called speech territory remain severely aphasic, but that, on the other hand, total recovery is seldom, if ever, seen.

Recent investigations by Bond and Brooks (1) reveal that the greater part of recovery of physical and mental functions in patients with severe head trauma occurs within the first six months after the injury. In the present material further improvement took place in several aphasics. Very slow, but gradual evolution from automatic to intellectual language was thus seen in a severely injured patient with a P.T.A. of at least 5 months (8). The patient received intensive logopedic treatment during the whole observation period of almost two years. It is worth mentioning that the patient first began to pay some attention to his verbal paraphasia more than a year after the trauma.

References

1. Bond, M. R. & Brooks, D. N.: Understanding the process of recovery as a basis for the investigation of rehabilitation for the brain injured. Scand J Rehab Med 8: 127, 1976.
2. Butfield, E. & Zangwill, O. L.: Reeducation in aphasia: A review of 70 cases. J Neurol Neurosurg Psychiat 9: 75, 1946.
3. Kertesz, A. & McCabe, P.: Recovery patterns and prognosis in aphasia. Brain 100: 1, 1977.
4. Schuell, H., Jenkins, J. J. & Jimenez-Pabon, E.: Aphasia in Adults. Harper & Row, New York, 1964.
5. Schuell, H.: Some dimensions of aphasic impairment in adults. Brit J Dis Com 1: 33, 1966.
6. Thomsen, I. V.: The patient with severe head injury and his family. Scand J Rehab Med 6: 180, 1974.
7. Thomsen, I. V.: Evaluation and outcome of aphasia in patients with severe closed head trauma. J Neurol Neurosurg Psychiat 38: 713, 1975.
8. Thomsen, I. V.: Evaluation and outcome of traumatic aphasia in patients with severe verified focal lesions. Folia Phoniat 28: 362, 1976.
9. Thomsen, I. V.: Verbal learning in aphasic and non-aphasic patients with severe head injuries. Scand J Rehab Med 9: 73, 1977.
10. Weisenburg, T. & McBride, K. E.: Aphasia. Commonwealth Fund, N.Y., 1935.
11. Wepman, J. M.: A conceptual model for the processes involved in recovery from aphasia. J Speech Hear Dis 18: 4, 1953.
12. Wepman, J. M.: Aphasia therapy: A new look. J Speech Hear Dis 37: 203, 1972.
13. Vignolo, L. A.: Evolution of aphasia and language rehabilitation: A retrospective exploratory study. Cortex 1: 344, 1964.

Cerebral lateralization of speech and singing after intracarotid amytal injection

H. M. BORCHGREVINK

Introduction

Speech and musical function apparently have a number of common features and corresponding elements. Both include the spectral analysis of complex sound duration (e.g. the recognition of vowels and chords) and the temporal analysis of sequential sound (e.g. the discrimination of phoneme combinations and rhythmic patterns).

From this point of view speech perception would not be expected to involve such unique psychological processes as has been proposed for instance by Lieberman (8). Hypothetically, one would rather assume that many of the so-called unique characteristics of speech perception also may be found in analogous psycho-acoustical functions as in musical perception. Besides, psycho-acoustical capacities required for speech processing would be expected to be present in individuals or species lacking our conventional language abilities.

Recent experimental findings support the reasoning presented above. Preverbal infants, with a mean age of only about 70 days, are capable of fairly complex rhythm discrimination and temporal grouping of sound analogous to what is required in language comprehension (4). So are certain birds (10). Music-like sounds are perceived categorically like phonemes (3). Musical intervals appear to be categorically perceived by musicians (2). Rats can discriminate between consonant and dissonant chord pairs (1)!

The promising rehabilitation effect of Melodic Intonation Therapy on aphasia (11) was regarded to be of interest from this point of view. It indicates that disturbed speech performance may be facilitated in some hitherto unknown way by the still intact musical abilities. In the case of unilateral brain pathology and aphasia it was assumed that this facilitation most probably would be due to cerebral processes in the unaffected non-dominant hemisphere, which is generally believed to control various musical functions including melody and pitch (5, 6, 7, 9). If so, one would expect to observe a corresponding interference between speech and musical functions upon selective dominant hemisphere anesthesia. Aiming at an improved understanding of the problem, the following experiment was performed.

Method

The relation between the capacities for speech (counting) and singing and their respective cerebral localization was investigated in three patients under selective anesthesia of one hemisphere after the other by Wada intracarotid amytal technique (12) (which was performed for diagnostic reasons). All suffered from left temporal epilepsy.

Patient 1 was a 14-year-old girl, intelligent, ambidextrous, musically trained (piano). Epilepsy after meningitis 10 months old.

Patient 2 was a 23-year-old woman, intellectually impaired, righthanded, very little musical training, living in institutions for the last 13 years. Epilepsy of unknown (familial) origin. Dysphasic.

Patient 3 was a 32-year-old man, intelligent, though slow and dysphasic (Broca's aphasia symptoms). Righthanded. Little musical training (local choir). Epilepsy caused by slow-growing fronto-temporal tumor in the left hemisphere.

Prior to the experiment the patients were instructed to count, to hum a part of a tune and (only patient 3) to count to this tune, repeating 1, 2, 3, 4, 5, 6, 7 as if this was the text of the tune. The tune chosen was the first four bars of the "Alle Vögel sind schon da", well known in its Norwegian version to all the patients, and being convenient for the purpose because of fairly distinct rhythm, starting and ending on the same note/pitch, and including both rising and falling major triad as well as the octave.

Immediately before the intracarotid Amytal injection a tape recording was made of each patient's counting and humming performance for the purpose of reference/control (Nagra IV Kudelski tape recorder and Kudelski microphone). 75 mg Amytal was injected on each side with some 30 min intermediate pause. This amount was sufficient to produce a short temporary hemiplegia in the patients. The patients were continuously asked to count, to hum or to do both simultaneously during the injections and/or during the phases of recovery while their performances were tape recorded. These recordings were compared to the reference recordings made prior to the injections. The following results are based on the judgements of musical listeners.

Results[1]

Patient 1

Right intracarotid injection while counting: she stopped counting at the moment of being hemiplegic. Repeated right intracarotid injection while humming the tune: the patient gradually lost tonal control, but preserved control of rhythm and could communicate verbally.

---

[1] The results were presented to the Symposium by tape-recordings.

Left intracarotid injection while counting: she stopped counting before being hemiplegic. During recovery the patient was unable to hum. 65 sec after the injection she counted normally, and she suddenly regained normal singing/ humming ability after 110 sec with full tonal and rhythmic control.

Patient 2

Right intracarotid injection while counting: she stopped counting at the moment of being hemiplegic. During recovery she smiled after 170 sec on being addressed, lifted left arm after 200 sec, was able to hum after 250 sec with impaired tonal control, but with preserved control of rhythm.

Left intracarotid injection while humming the tune: there was gradually increasing loss of rhythmic distinction but with preserved tonality, appro- aching "glissando". During recovery she was unable to speak, count and hum. 80 sec after the injection she was asked verbally to sing with no response, but started to hum when the investigator hummed the tune. Her tonal control was unaffected while rhythmic distinction was poor. Rhythmic control was gradually regained. When asked to count, she hummed. Then the investigator counted to the tune, and occasional digits appeared in her humming (115 sec after the injection). After 150 sec she replied "yes" and counted a couple of digits with perseveration. Then she started to count to the melody. For the following minute she was able to count fluently with melody, but could hardly count at all without melody.

Patient 3

Right intracarotid injection while counting to the melody: he preserved counting ability and rhythm while gradually losing tonal control until the melody was not recognizable. During recovery he first counted monotonously with preserved rhythm (55 sec after the injection). After 115 sec he regained increasing tonal control and counted to normally controlled melody after 230 sec.

Left intracarotid injection while counting to the melody: he suddenly stopped both counting and singing after 45 sec before being hemiplegic. 85 sec after the injection he gradually regained the ability to speak, could count monotonously with perseverations after 235 sec and was suddenly able to sing and count after 370 sec with good control of tonality and rhythm. After 410 sec he was able to hum without counting.

Discussion

In all three patients speech was located in the left hemisphere according to conventional Wada criteria (12).

In patient 2 singing facilitated counting upon dominant (left) hemisphere anesthesia. This indicates that the psychological mechanism behind the effect of Melodic Intonation Therapy most likely is located in the nondominant hemisphere. If so, the facilitation observed in this therapy for aphasia might not be a facilitation in the sense of restoring the function in normal pathways of speech.

Rather, the mechanism might imply an elimination of the blocked parts of the impaired pathways in the dominant hemisphere by using alternative routes in the non-dominant hemisphere being available by melodic performance. It might be a limited "detour" into the non-dominant hemisphere, the function resting largely upon dominant pathways, or alternatively imply activation of potential speech pathways in the non-dominant hemisphere to the extent of a total neglect of the dominant hemisphere pathways. In either case, therapy for aphasia might rather concentrate on establishing speech function by stimulating the most often unaffected non-dominant hemisphere, for instance by way of musical function, which may be intact even in "total" aphasia. Investigations aiming to illuminate the relation between speech and musical functions in patients with aphasia have been initiated by the author at a clinical center for aphasia in Oslo.

All three patients lost tonal control of singing during non-dominant (right) hemisphere anesthesia, supporting earlier reports (5, 6, 7, 9). Contrary to what has been reported (6, 9), rhythm was preserved in all three patients upon non-dominant hemisphere anesthesia. Besides, patient 2 showed extensive lack of rhythmic distinction in her "glissando" singing upon dominant (left) hemisphere anesthesia. Rhythm thus appears to be con- trolled by the dominant hemisphere, which is consistent with the fact that rhythm requires temporal analysis of sequential sound, as does speech per- ception. This may explain the more extensive cerebral lateralization of chords than of melodies in dichotic listening tests reported by Gordon (5) as melodies consist of both tonal and rhythmic elements, while chords only contain tonal elements.

Upon dominant (left) hemisphere anesthesia, patient 3 simultaneously stopped counting and singing abruptly. He gradually regained speaking and counting ability. Then fully controlled singing appeared to be "released" facilitated by counting. During recovery from dominant (left) hemisphere anesthesia in patient 1 counting ability was correspondingly restored before the sudden "release" of normal singing. This indicates that in these two patients the act of starting to sing was in some way blocked by the anesthetized dominant hemisphere, while tonal control capacity was preserved by the un- affected non-dominant hemisphere without being "put through". The same mechanism might explain why patient 3, who had a mild degree of Broca's aphasia due to tumor in the left fronto-temporal region, had problems of ini- tiating singing as well as speech performance prior to anesthesia. As stated above, all three patients lost tonal control upon non-dominant (right) hemi- sphere anesthesia. They were, however, still able to sing. One may therefore conclude that in some individuals the expressive act of singing is controlled by the dominant (left) hemisphere in spite of the precise control of tonality and pitch being located in the non-dominant (right) hemisphere.

One must bear in mind that the cerebral pathology of these patients may have influenced their cerebral dominance for several functions. Patient 1 was ambidextrous, eating with one hand and writing with the other. However, they all had speech located in the left hemisphere according to Wada criteria.

If the above findings are reproducible in a larger patient series, the relevance of a therapeutic approach in aphasia through musical functions and/or other modes of non-dominant hemisphere stimulation is obvious. Tests for musical abilities then ought to be a part of the diagnosis of aphasia, aiding the therapist's efforts in finding "peep-holes through the patient's speech barricade". This might lead to more specific and thus more adequate individual therapy.

Conclusion

There is a close, but complex, connection between speech and musical function. Both apparently consist of a multitude of subfunctions, many of which rely upon common psychological mechanisms. This implies extensive possibilities of interference between the two functions, weakening the concepts of distinct cerebral dominance for speech and music. Each subfunction may nevertheless be distinctively lateralized. This indicates the relevance of a musical approach in the therapy of speech disorders like aphasia.

Tonal and pitch control was found to be lateralized to the non-dominant (right) hemisphere. However, the results indicate that rhythm is controlled by the dominant (left) hemisphere, which also controls the initiation of singing as well as speech in some individuals.

The experiment showed that singing may facilitate speech and vice versa, both upon dominant (left) hemisphere anesthesia. This indicates that the effect of Melodic Intonation Therapy on aphasia is due to psychological processes in the non-dominant (right) hemisphere. Accordingly, the therapeutic approach in aphasia might preferably imply non-dominant (right) hemisphere stimulation by for instance music.

References

1. Borchgrevink, H. M.: Musical chord preferences in man elucidated by animal experiments. Paper presented at the IV Int Congr Europ Assoc Audiophon Centers, Vejle, Denmark, 1976.
2. Borchgrevink, H. M. (in prep.): Categorical perception of musical intervals. Report.
3. Cutting, J. E. & Rosner, B. S.: Perceptual categories for musiclike sounds: Implications for theories of speech perception. Quart J Exp Psychol 28: 361, 1976.
4. Demany, L., McKenzie, B. & Vurpillot, E.: Rythm perception in early infancy. Nature 266: 718, 1977.

5. Gordon, H. W.: Hemispheric asymmetry and musical performance. Science 189: 68, 1975.
6. Gordon, H. W. & Bogen, J. E.: Hemispheric lateralization of singing after intracarotid sodium amylobarbitone. J Neurol Neurosurg Psychiat 37: 727, 1974.
7. Kimura, D.: Left-right differences in the perception of melodies. Quart J Exp Psychol 16: 355, 1964.
8. Lieberman, A. M.: Some characteristics of perception in the speech mode. Perception and its disorders 48: 238, 1970.
9. Milner, B.: Laterality effects in audition. In: Mountcastle (ed.), Interhemispheric Relations and Cerebral Dominance. Baltimore, 1962.
10. Reinert, J.: Takt- und Rhythmusunterscheidung bei Dohlen. Z. Tierpsychol 22: 668 (summary), 1965.
11. Sparks, R. W. & Holland, A. L.: Method: Melodic intonation therapy for aphasia. J Speech Hear Disord 41: 287, 1976.
12. Wada, J. & Rasmussen, T.: Intracarotid injection of sodium amytal for the lateralization of cerebral speech dominance. J Neurosurg 17: 266, 1960.

Psychiatric problems in aphasia

D. FRANK BENSON

Aphasia is both common and serious and has obvious psychiatric complications. Despite a century of intense study of aphasia, however, relatively little attention has been given to the psychiatric aspects of the disorder. This presentation will focus on the psychiatric considerations that affect the course of aphasia.

For clarity, the subject will be separated into four divisions. The divisions are not mutually exclusive and a considerable overlap of psychiatric problems is standard. For ease of discussion, however, the following topics will be presented separately: 1) the psychosocial aspects of aphasia; 2) the neuro-behavioral aspects of aphasia; 3) the intelligence and competency aspects of aphasia; 4) the psychiatric aspects of aphasia rehabilitation.

Before outlining the psychiatric considerations, some background information concerning aphasia is warranted. Aphasia may be defined as the loss or impairment of language caused by brain damage. Language can be considered that exclusively human capability of placing ideas and thoughts into a set of symbols that can be communicated to and understood by other humans and, as such, language can be separated from both speech and thought. It is the loss of this function, language, that is called aphasia.

How common is aphasia? This question is unanswerable until sufficient statistics have been gathered but approximately 40% of cerebral vascular accidents cause some interference with language (between 250,000 and 500,000 CVAs occur annually in the United States alone). In addition, aphasia can be the result of trauma, brain tumor, complications of neurosurgery and less frequent causes such as the degenerative diseases, infectious diseases, etc. A sizeable number of individuals sustain greater or lesser degrees of language disturbance annually and, as most survive the initial insult, a large ever growing reservoir of aphasic individuals is produced. At present, most cases of aphasia seen clinically result from vascular accidents. Historically, however, war-induced brain trauma has been a major cause of language disturbance and the increasing prevalence of serious head trauma in traffic accidents suggests that there will be an increasing number of trauma-induced aphasic conditions in the future.

Aphasia from CVA almost invariably has an acute and totally unexpected

Supported in part by funds from grant NS06209 from the National Institutes of Health to the Boston University School of Medicine and in part by Research funds from the Veterans Administration.

onset and the aphasia of head trauma has a similarly sudden onset. The acute, unanticipated onset is an important psychiatric feature of aphasia. Against this background we can examine four major aspects—the psychosocial, the neurobehavioral, the intellectual and the psychiatric aspects of aphasia therapy itself.

Psychosocial aspects

Probably the single most important psychosocial factor in most cases of aphasia revolves about the sudden, calamitous alteration of lifestyle caused by the disorder. In addition to the loss of language, similarly drastic alterations in employment status, social and family position and recreational opportunities suddenly disappear.

Alteration of economic status is a factor of concern for many aphasics. Most become aphasic at the prime of their earning capacity, at a time when they are comparatively independent and self-caring. With the onset of aphasia this capability suddenly disappears and, with awareness of the new status, many aphasics eventually realize that the loss of economic independence will be permanent.

Coupled with the drastic deterioration of economic status, is a similar alteration in the individual's position in society. By the time in life when aphasia occurs, most individuals have established strong patterns in both work and social activities. Relationships have been developed with employees, co-workers, neighbors, recreation associates and others, a status that is abruptly changed with the onset of aphasia. Realization of the degree of social change occurs slowly for most aphasics, but eventually becomes an important psychosocial consideration.

In a similar vein, most aphasics must eventually face an alteration of position in the family. If the degree of aphasia is comparatively mild, the patient may retain much of the prior status within the family but if the degree of language disturbance is sufficiently severe, the spouse or other members of the family must assume much of the leadership role. Thus, aphasic individuals suddenly find themselves in a passive, child-like position within their own family. Many aphasics react violently by directing negative hostile, paranoid and downright cruel behavior toward close family members. Again, realization is not immediate and can be intelligently and carefully managed by some families so as to minimize the loss. Many families, however, are not capable of gracefully effecting this alteration. If, instead of offering support, the spouse expresses anger and hostility based on new responsibilities, a serious psychological problem is added to the aphasic's list of troubles. A change of position within the family affects most aphasics and must be recognized as a significant psychological factor in their disability.

In addition, the aphasic often suffers a serious alteration in physical capability. The previously active, self-caring individual may be hemiparetic, must relearn standing and walking, and can never again participate in athletics and many other previously enjoyed physical activities.

Yet another psychosocial aspect which must be faced eventually is the real or imagined loss of sexual capability. Aphasia, itself, does not interfere with sexual powers, but major degrees of paralysis and the inability to communicate accurately may act as a considerable hindrance to normal sexual relationships. Many aphasics suspect that they will never regain normal sexual activities, another adjustment problem of major importance to many aphasics.

Based on the many losses noted above, there is a natural tendency for the aphasic to enter into a grief reaction. There can be a true grief for the individual physical and social losses but, in addition, the combined losses may produce a serious disturbance of self-image. When the amount of loss is severe (or the premorbid self-image was precarious), an overwhelming feeling of self-deprecation and worthlessness, a reactive depression, may result. Such feelings do not develop immediately but build up over an extended period following the onset of aphasia.

While reactive depression is common, it is far from universal. In fact, the naive observer would anticipate that disorders of self-image should be greater than is apparent in most aphasic patients. Often this discrepancy reflects the degree of mental deterioration caused by the brain injury rather than the product of an intrinsic ego strength.

Aphasics with reactive depression sink deeply within themselves. They often stop eating, refuse social interaction with therapists, other patients and even family members, and exhibit a passive non-cooperation. The time of onset of reactive depression following onset of aphasia is quite variable. Some aphasics enter this state rapidly but most show a delay of weeks or even months before the grief reaction sets in. In general, reactive depression can be considered a healthy sign, indicating that the patient has recovered sufficient intellectual competence to recognize the severity of the problem and the drastic alterations in lifestyle. With this more realistic state, rehabilitation measures can be more problem oriented and are more likely to be successful. Reactive depression, however, is an extremely painful disturbance, both for the patients and those who deal with them. When handled correctly reactive depressions are usually short-lived but demand careful attention.

Neurobehavioral aspects

In addition to the psychosocial aspects, important alterations of emotional response are noted which apparently depend on the location of the brain lesion. The significance of behavioral abnormalities based on focal pathology has been recognized only recently and future studies will probably produce clearer delineation of focal anatomical and physiological influences on the psychological responses. At present, aphasic patients can be divided into two large groups, those with fluent verbal output and those with a non-fluent expressive disorder. Recent experimental work has demonstrated specific anatomical correlations underlying the two variations in verbal output. Almost without exception, fluent, paraphasic output occurs only when the pathology is located posterior to the fissure of Rolando. Conversely, almost all non-fluent aphasics have pathology involving the frontal lobe, anterior to the fissure of Rolando.

Two distinctly different behavioral responses to aphasia can be correlated with the two varieties of aphasia and, thus, with the location of the aphasia producing lesion. Non-fluent aphasics are usually aware, at least to some degree, of their new problems and tend to become depressed. In addition, they often know exactly what they want to say but find they cannot say it, an extremely frustrating situation. Many patients with nonfluent aphasia show both depression and frustration. Both conditions are potentially serious and, occurring in combination, tend to aggravate each other. If a patient with these problems is not handled carefully during periods of severe frustration, another, far more serious problem, called the catastrophic reaction, can occur. If non-fluent aphasics are repeatedly asked to perform simple verbal tasks that formerly would have been accomplished readily but cannot be done now, they can become angry, hostile and negative and develop an emotional breakdown with loud crying, withdrawal, extreme negativity and widespread hostility. Such patients may stop eating and caring for themselves and may arbitrarily refuse to communicate for days at a time. During a catastrophic reaction the patient will refuse to talk or listen to individuals who were previously of importance, including members of the hospital staff and their own family. The sleep pattern, diet and personal hygiene are altered and the patient must be considered dangerously ill. Most catastrophic reactions are short-lived, sometimes lasting only a few hours but at other times continuing for several days. The best treatment is prophylactic: the frustrated, depressed, anterior aphasic should never be pushed hard in language tasks. Continual failure is unpleasant for everyone and much more so for the unfortunate aphasic who knows the correct response but finds it locked in. If a catastrophic reaction does take place, the major treatment is empathy and concern. This, plus the healing quality of time, eventually proves successful. But, if aphasic patients are handled correctly, particularly not pushed in routine language testing, the catastrophic reaction will not occur.

The depression of anterior aphasia must always be considered a serious problem. Suicide is occasionally feared in some non-fluent patients and must be accepted as a real possibility. It has not been our experience, however, that these patients represent a serious suicidal risk. In particular, early recognition of depressive changes and appropriate management can successfully combat the depression of the anterior aphasic. As an example, a 22-year-old brain injured soldier with a right hemiplegia and anterior aphasia became acutely depressed when a girlfriend politely but firmly let him know that she was not interested in marriage to a crippled person. The resulting depression complicated the considerable frustrations of his physical and language disorders and produced a worrisome situation. Ward personnel were alerted, both to beware of suicidal attempts and to offer extra attempts at interrelationship. The process was successful in that he recovered from the depths of grief in only a few days and returned to active therapy efforts.

The psychiatric problems noted in fluent aphasia are strikingly different. In the first place, many individuals with fluent paraphasic aphasia have a major problem comprehending spoken language. They are often unaware of their comprehension deficit and, in many instances, lack concern. This combination, unawareness and unconcern, stands in sharp contrast to the frustrated, depressed condition of the anterior aphasic. Patients with posterior aphasia who cannot monitor their own verbal output fail to realize that their jargon output is incomprehensible. If a tape recording is made of this output and played back, many fluent paraphasic patients will deny that it is their own voice. Possibly because of the unawareness of their own comprehension disturbance, posterior aphasics have a tendency to blame communication difficulties on others. They may suggest that others are not talking clearly enough to be understood and/or not paying sufficient attention to what the patient is saying. They may believe that persons they see talking together (but cannot understand) are using a special code and talking about them. This amounts to a paranoia, similar to the well recognized paranoia of acquired deafness. In addition, some posterior aphasics show a tendency for impulsive behavior. The combination of paranoia and impulsiveness may make such patients dangerous to themselves and others. Physical attacks against medical personnel, family members, other patients or themselves can occur. Almost all aphasic patients who need custodial type psychiatric management are posterior aphasics with poor comprehension, unawareness of their deficit, paranoia and impulsive behavior.

In addition to these two striking psychiatric responses, a number of additional neurobehavioral problems may be seen in the aphasic. These disorders are numerous, common and further complicate many aphasic disturbances. Because of space limitations only a few of these neurobehavioral disorders can be outlined here; any one of them can be of critical importance for an individual aphasic.

For example, a common behavioral complication is the presence of confusion. Confusional states are frequent in medical practice, sometimes following structural damage to the brain but more often are drug induced or caused by metabolic abnormalities. The patient in a confusional state has difficulty maintaining a coherent line of thought and verbal responses are liable to be abnormal. While language output, per se, is usually adequate, the number of meaningful substantive words is often decreased and frequent, unexpected changes in topic make the conversation difficult to follow. When a confusional state complicates aphasia, the combined product is often that of an overwhelming aphasic disturbance. Much of the apparent language problem may clear, however, if the confusional state is recognized and treated appropriately.

Another neurobehavioral condition complicating many cases of aphasia is decreased motivation, the presence of apathy or inertia. Traditionally, this state is thought to result from damage to the frontal lobes but probably occurs more frequently with subcortical pathology. Aphasics with a significant degree of apathy are poor candidates for aphasia therapy and unlikely to make a good spontaneous recovery unless the apathy clears. There is a strong tendency to blame the patient for the poor motivation and the subsequently limited recovery. That the patient's lack of motivation interferes with therapy is certainly true but almost invariably, the apathy is based on neurological damage and is beyond the control of the patient. In some cases it is amenable to specific treatment, however.

The possibility that an aphasic has a memory disturbance (amnesia) deserves consideration. Amnesia is an uncommon complication of middle cerebral artery occlusion, the type of stroke most often leading to aphasia. There is, however, a recognized amnesic stroke disorder that follows involvement of the posterior cerebral arteries. Many aphasic individuals have disease involving multiple cerebral vessels and the possibility of amnesia complicating aphasia must be considered. Amnesia is much more common as a complicating factor in the aphasia caused by brain trauma. In fact, amnesia is the most common residual of brain trauma and if aphasia has also been produced, the two are likely to coexist. Amnesia is a serious complication in individuals with aphasia because the presence of an inability to learn almost totally obviates any potential for successful aphasia therapy. Language therapy must await improvement in the amnesia and this may or may not occur.

Another neurobehavioral complication is a true dementia—a serious impairment of intellectual functions. Vascular disease can, by itself, produce a dementia, particularly if there have been multiple infarctions involving different areas of both hemispheres. An acute aphasia may complicate a degenerative type of dementia such as Alzheimer's disease; similarly, brain trauma can damage the brain in many areas and a combination of aphasia and dementia is a common complication of trauma. The presence of dementia seriously decreases the possibility of successful aphasia therapy.

One type of aphasia, global aphasia, is extremely resistant to language therapy. By simple definition, global aphasia refers to an almost total loss of both verbal output and the comprehension of spoken language. Many attempts to treat global aphasia have proved unsuccessful and a number of aphasia therapists suggest that global aphasia cannot be significantly altered by therapy. One postulated explanation for the failure of global aphasics to respond, even to intense language therapy, concerns bilateral brain damage. It is surmised that a compromised right hemisphere cannot participate in the recovery of communication. Whether this theory is correct remains controversial but it is true that many individuals with global aphasia do not respond to conventional forms of aphasia therapy.

Finally, a serious complication which may or may not be based on specific neurobehavioral disorder deserves attention. This is the possibility of suicide. Some aphasic patients do commit suicide and this possibility of suicide must be considered seriously, particularly in posterior aphasics. As noted earlier, depression, frustration and the catastrophic reaction occur primarily in the anterior or non-fluent aphasic, a combination that would appear ominous but individuals with this type of aphasia rarely threaten suicide. In caring for over 2 000 aphasics we have never had an anterior aphasic attempt suicide. Actually, suicide is rare in all types of aphasia but apparently occurs more frequently in the posterior, fluent aphasic who is both paranoid and impulsive. As such individuals become aware of the seriousness and probable permanence of their disability and the alterations in lifestyle that will result, the possibility of an impulsive self-destructive act must be considered. To say the least, treatment of the suicide potential in these patients is difficult. The inability to communicate caused by the posterior aphasia removes most of the person-to-person, psychotherapeutic measures usually advised. Similarly, most aphasics cannot talk out their problems. Obviously, standard suicide precautions should be maintained and, in addition to removal of potential suicidal devices, considerable effort should be made to establish interpersonal relationships and minimize frustrations. Even when the suicide potentiality is recognized and appropriate measures are taken, a well planned life ending act can occur. Management of such patients is a tremendous burden and must be shared by all who are in contact with them.

Intelligence and legal competency

There has long been discussion concerning the effect of aphasia on intelligence. Many experts have suggested that language is such an integral part of intelligence that all aphasics must suffer at least some degree of intellectual deterioration. Other experts insist that many retain derogatory diagnosis of dementia on all aphasic patients. Intelligence itself is a difficult concept and testing for intelligence in aphasia is hampered because most standardized tests rely heavily on verbal instructions and/or responses. Most I.Q. tests are severely limited as tools for assessing the intelligence of an aphasic. The performance section of the Wechsler Adult Intelligence Scale, appropriately interpolated, does offer some evidence of residual intelligence and many aphasics, including some with severe language loss, score in a near normal range. Even a decrease in the performance part of the WAIS, however, may only reflect the severity of the aphasia, as several of the performance items also depend upon language skills and may be artificially depressed. On the other hand, there can be little doubt that many aphasics do suffer a significant decrease in intellectual competency and in some this disturbance is rather obvious. Each aphasic must be judged independently, utilizing whatever tools are available; the evaluation of an individual aphasic's residual intelligence is best determined by the personal judgment of an experienced examiner.

The ability of aphasic individuals to manage their own affairs frequently comes into question. Obviously, legal and business affairs demanding high level language skills, such as the reading or writing of contracts and mortgages cannot be performed by severely aphasic individuals. The question often rises however, as to whether aphasics are competent to make decisions concerning management of their own funds, future housing, sale of property or investments and, most difficult of all, in the making of a will. Each aphasic must be judged individually. Without question, many aphasic individuals are competent to manage their own affairs and deserve the protection of a conservator or guardian. There is a third group, those with distinct disability but who, with appropriate help, can make many of their own major decisions. This group is difficult to evaluate and can produce serious controversy. As far as possible patients in this group should be given considerable help in an attempt to keep them in control of their own affairs.

Psychiatric aspects of aphasia rehabilitation

Treatment of the aphasic patient is a complex task that must include attention to potential psychiatric complications and take advantage of any psychological support that can be made available. Most aphasics also have some degree of physical disability that needs special therapy. Even partial recovery of physical competency has a positive psychological effect and therapists in physical medicine and related fields should emphasize all successes during the treatment of aphasics. Most hemiplegic aphasics can eventually be returned to independent walking. The resulting independence produces a tremendous boost to the patient's image and should be actively promoted. Success in physical activities can be an effective antidote for some of the psychiatric complications of aphasia.

In a similar manner, language therapy should be a positive psychological factor. Even if the patient makes only small gains in language, improvement in the ability to communicate is valuable and all improvements should be emphasized to the patient. In the past much aphasia therapy has been directed at this type of psychosocial support and, in the opinion of many, remains a major contribution of aphasia therapy.

Outlining of long term goals has proved rather difficult in the treatment of many aphasics. Unlike physical disability which tends to stabilize, language dysfunction may continue improving over a period of several years. Nonetheless, long term goals should be established for the aphasic patient. Some patients will fall short of their goal but this is less important than their attempts toward reaching the goal. Eventually all aphasics plateau in active language therapy but this stage does not indicate that improvement has ceased. If placed in a favorable environment, particularly one where they are encouraged to communicate, many aphasics continue to improve in language ability over a prolonged span of time.

If possible, it is well to have the aphasic patient participate in group activities with other aphasics. In the group the aphasic can try out his limited communication capabilities on a uniquely sympathetic audience and under the guidance of an experienced therapist. At the onset, the aphasic feels isolated; joining a group who suffer the same disorder decreases the sense of isolation. In addition, other aphasics are noted whose problems were as bad or worse than the patients but who have improved considerably. Similarly, some patients in the group will have even greater problems than the patient. Both observations tend to bolster the patient's self image. Participation in a group demands interpersonal relationships. Most aphasics are limited in social interaction and, while their participation may appear negligible, particularly at first, reacting in a group may decrease this problem.

Several psychiatric complications that may appear during the period of rehabilitation demand specific treatment. Reactive depression is a healthy psychic phenomenon for the recovering aphasic and, within limits, should be allowed to run its course. During this period, extra amounts of sympathy and attention are rewarded with a more rapid recovery. Following recovery from a reactive depression, the aphasic usually shows improved participation in rehabilitation activities.

The neurobehavioral complications of the anterior or non-fluent aphasic may need specific treatment. Certainly a great deal of emotional support, encouragement and understanding during the period of extreme depression and frustration are indicated. Not to be forgotten is that the aphasic comprehends better than he expresses; rehabilitation personnel should never talk about the patient in his presence as though he were not competent to understand. Caution in not pushing the examination of the anterior aphasic too far in testing is valuable. If anterior aphasics suffer long standing and serious depression, particularly if there is a history of previous depressive problems, treatment with anti-depressant drugs may be indicated. The major physical treatments of depression such as large doses of the anti-depressant medications or electroshock therapy are usually unnecessary. In general, the more supportive types of therapy, such as that offered by the language therapist, the physical therapist, the nursing staff, the physicians and particularly the family are effective in helping the anterior aphasic cope with his new life.

Psychiatric problems of posterior aphasics are much more difficult to handle. These patients do not fully understand what is being said, may not be aware of their own problems and may even show a true anosognosia, a denial of their own aphasic problems. If such a patient becomes agitated or seriously paranoid, the use of strong tranquilizers, such as the phenothiazines, is indicated and placement in a custodial or locked-ward situation may be necessary during periods of intense agitation. Even during periods of agitation, however, attempts at active language rehabilitation therapy should be continued.

The occurrence of reactive depression in posterior aphasia is encouraging, indicating a realization of the problem and a better potential for active rehabilitation. On the other hand, the onset of depression plus continued impulsiveness can make these patients potentially dangerous. All psychiatric problems of the posterior aphasic are potentially serious and demand careful management.

Obviously the support techniques offered by the rehabilitation team are forms of psychotherapy but the use of formal psychiatric therapy in the aphasic patient deserves comment because special approaches are required. Most contemporary psychiatrists communicate with their patients almost exclusively by verbal exchange and they find it both difficult and frustrating to work with aphasics. It is usually better for the psychiatrist to work through an experienced speech pathologist. The speech pathologist, specifically trained and competent in dealing with the aphasic, can maintain communication and the psychiatrist should function as an advisor or supervisor rather than as the active therapist. It is well to discuss the psychiatric problems of the aphasic with members of the family and encourage them, as much as possible, to include the patient in family activities and planning. By using all available approaches, most psychiatric complications of aphasia can be managed successfully.

Communication aids
for speech disabled:
Trends for international cooperation

OLLE HÖÖK

At the present time persons with impaired speech capacity on the basis of central nervous system pathology (anarthria–dysarthria) have very limited access to technical aids that may compensate for their communication handicap.

A few years ago a 22-year-old woman was referred to the Institute of Rehabilitation Medicine in Gothenburg. A few months earlier she had sustained a serious traffic accident with a severe brain stem contusion which rendered her unconscious and on a respirator for two months. She was practically wheelchair bound due to bilateral pyramidal tract lesions and had ataxia and anarthria. In spite of her brain damage her intellectual capacity was rather good.

In order to increase the possibility for her communication in spite of anarthria and ataxia, an apparatus was designed which fulfilled the following requirements:

1. It could be used even when communicating in a group of persons, i.e. the letters that she selected should be seen simultaneously by the patient as well as by several others.
2. It was so small that it could be mounted on an ordinary wheelchair table.
3. The key-board was designed in such a way that if the patient's hand inadvertently fell on it, the keys would not be pushed down by mistake.

Such an electronic writing device with a key-board and display screens was constructed (3). Similar devices are now available on the market (6).

In Sweden (8.2 million inhabitants) we estimate that patients with anarthria or severe dysarthria for whom such aids would be of great importance, comprise a group of about 1,000 persons (1 : 8 000). There are also in Sweden about 100 school-children with serious speech difficulties in spite of normal intelligence.

The design and selection of technical aids requires that they be constructed according to the patient's physical and psychosocial profile, i.e. the aid must be chosen in close cooperation between patient, medical officer and technician.

In order to develop improved communication aids, the Swedish Institute for the Handicapped in Stockholm in collaboration with the International

Table I. *Swedish steering committee for developing technical aids for the speech impaired*

I. *Phoniatry*
    Phoniatric Clinic, Huddinge Hospital, Huddinge
    Björn Fritzell, Chief physician
    Britta Hammarberg, Speech therapist
    Folke Bernadotte-hemmet, Uppsala
    Gunnel Thunell, Speech therapist

II. *Rehabilitation Medicine + Habilitation*
    Inst. of Rehabilitation Medicine, University of Göteborg, Göteborg
    Olle Höök, Professor & Chairman
    Bräcke Östergård Habilitation Centre, Göteborg
    Ingemar Olow, Chief physician
    Swedish Centre for Special Communication Aids, Bräcke Östergård, Göteborg
    Ulf Lekemo, Director

III. *Technology*
    Inst. for Speech Transmission, Royal Inst. of Technology, Stockholm
    Gunnar Fant, Professor & Chairman
    Arne Risberg, Civ.engineer
    Karoly Galyas, Civ.engineer

IV. *Linguistics*
    Inst. of Linguistics, University of Stockholm, Stockholm
    Björn Lindblom, Professor & Chairman

V. *The Swedish Institute for the Handicapped, Stockholm*
    Birger Roos, Techn. Director
    Margita Lundman, Psychologist
    Mette Granström, B. A., ICTA
    Elisabeth Tenenholtz, Speech therapist

VI. *Swedish Association for Handicapped*
    The Central Committee of Organizations of and for the handicapped, Stockholm
    Rolf Utberg, Office manager

VII. *Funds*
    The Swedish Board for Technical Development, Stockholm
    Hans-Göran Karlsson, Head of Section for Social Techniques
    Gösta Lagerman, Chief engineer

Commission on Technical Aids, Housing and Transportation (ICTA) initiated a special project three years ago.

A steering committee of experts from various fields of knowledge such as technicians for speech transmission, specialists in phoniatry, linguistics, doctors working with neurological rehabilitation and habilitation has been guiding the project from its beginning (Table I).

We have also had discussions with many individuals and groups in other countries. Especially we will mention Luster and Vanderheiden's reports (5). A survey on international research and development projects for technical aids for the speech impaired has been compiled (4).

Table II. *Technical aids in patients with speech disturbances*

Letter (pointing) plate
Motorized letter plate
Motorized letter-pushing device
Electronic communication device with display
  (a) without letter memory
  (b) with letter memory
Keyboard with presentation of the letters on a television screen
Keyboard with presentation of the written word for speech in a computerized monitor
Voice amplifier

Within the Swedish group different technical aids have been constructed: from very simple aids such as rotating wheels with letters or pictures or simple sentences to those dependent on sophisticated computers which generate synthesized speech (Table II).

In cooperation with our Habilitation Centre in Göteborg an investigation is now going on which has resulted in a detailed classification of different speech disturbances as well as the patient's physical, psychic and social status (Table III).

The following example of work carried out at Bräcke Östergård Habilitation Center in Göteborg serves to illustrate an individual case. A 15 year old boy with dystonia, athetoid dyscoordination, and anarthria was given the opportunity to try a communication machine, which produced synthesized speech. The instrument was constructed at the Royal Technical Institute in Stockholm by Fant and his group (1).

Two computer terminals have been placed in Göteborg with the keyboards connected to the telephone line to the Stockholm computer. The terminals could be located at any place. At present one is kept by the patient and one with his comrade.

The boy has been highly stimulated by using this device. He has tried to communicate, even with his old letter-plate and similar simpler aids, with family members and teachers in a more vivid and interested way than before. Also his family has been tremendously stimulated and there is evidence of greater interest in the boy's communication problems.

Although this type of communication machine is still rather large in a few years period it is likely that it can be reduced to a size that will make it portable and perhaps may be located on a wheelchair.

In 1976 the Swedish Government Commission on Handicapped Persons published a report entitled: "Culture for Everybody". As a result of this report the Swedish parliament has decided that better technical aids should be developed and distributed to those with language deficits, by rather generous state grants.

There is considerable heterogenity amongst those with severe speech dys-

Table III. *Factors to be considered when choosing appropriate technical aids*

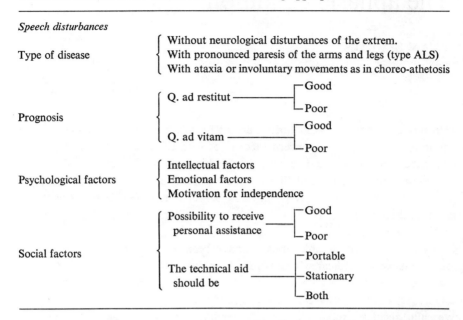

Speech disturbances

Type of disease	Without neurological disturbances of the extrem. With pronounced paresis of the arms and legs (type ALS) With ataxia or involuntary movements as in choreo-athetosis
Prognosis	Q. ad restitut — Good / Poor Q. ad vitam — Good / Poor
Psychological factors	Intellectual factors Emotional factors Motivation for independence
Social factors	Possibility to receive personal assistance — Good / Poor The technical aid should be — Portable / Stationary / Both

functions. They vary with respect to the type of motor problem, degree of residual functional motor control, basic intelligence, cognitive abilities and emotional-motivational status. Because of this, no single communication device can be considered uniformly applicable.

We also know, that the speech pathologist must do careful follow-up studies in order to monitor communication system needs relative to changes in the patient's status.

I would like to close with the words, that even when dealing with persons with aphasia *combined* with dysarthria, the potential for improving communication by technical aids should be kept in mind.

References

1. Fant, G., Galyas, K., Branderud, P., Svensson, S.-G. & McAllister, R.: Aids for speech-handicapped. Scand J Rehab Med 8: 65, 1976.
2. Höök, O.: Speech disturbance. Medical-Technical Aspects. Scand J Rehab Med 8: 55, 1976.
3. Lindberg, B. & Höök, O.: Communication aids for patients with anarthria. Scand J Rehab Med 6: 102, 1974.
4. Lundman, Margita: Technical aids for the speech impaired—a survey. The Swedish Institute for the Handicapped, Stockholm, 1977.
5. Luster, M. J. & Vanderheiden, G. C.: Annotated Bibliography of Communication Aids. Cerebral Palsy Communication Group, University of Wisconsin, Madison, Wisconsin 53706, USA, 1974.
6. Newell, A. F. & Brumfitt, P. J.: "Talking Brooch", communication aid. In: K. Copeland (ed.), pp. 104–108. Sector Publishing Limited, London, 1974.

The aphasic condition

YVAN LEBRUN

No sooner was aphasiology born than the founders of this branch of medicine quite logically began to concern themselves with the rehabilitation of aphasic patients. In his celebrated paper of 1865, which laid the foundation of cerebral dominance for speech, Paul Broca expressed the view that although complete recovery from aphasia may be difficult to achieve, intensive and prolonged speech therapy is likely to bring about considerable improvement in the patient's condition.

Ever since, innumerable aphasics have been given speech therapy. Under the guidance of dedicated professionals or resourceful and perseverative lay people, some of these patients have to a great extent regained their linguistic skills. Actress Patricia Neal, who was rendered severely aphasic by a cerebrovascular accident, recovered most of her language power thanks to the concerted efforts of her friends and the zeal and imagination of Val Griffith, a former beauty parlor attendant (6). Although other aphasics have not been able to regain much of their faculty of speech, many have made a remarkable adjustment to handicap, so that they can lead a near-normal life despite their language impairment. Zangwill (in Lebrun and Hoops, 11, p. 91–92) reported the case of the manager of a small radio and television business, who at 42 sustained a relatively severe mixed aphasia secondary to a left middle cerebral artery thrombosis. After a course of rehabilitation, he secured a job considerably less important than his previous one, but within a year was offered a responsible post in the sales department of a large glass manufactory. In this position he had to demonstrate great technical and commercial expertise and make judgments presupposing highly specialized knowledge and skill. Yet, this patient continued to show marked language defects, both expressive and receptive. He nonetheless managed his work without undue difficulty, apart from the use of the telephone, which he had to delegate to his secretary.

In many cases of aphasia, however, recovery and adjustment have been minimal, despite the efforts of both the patient and his speech therapist. In a number of instances this failure is due no doubt to the severity and extent of the cerebral lesion. In other cases, one cannot help thinking that the therapeutic approach has not been adequate. Moreover, the attitude of the patient's relatives may have slowed down, or even impeded, recovery or adjustment. To be sure, aphasia is often a baffling condition, with "tortuous, unexpected, deceptive qualities", to use the words of Helen Wulf (18), herself a post-stroke aphasic. No wonder therefore that the speech therapist should occasionally be at his wit's end and that the family should sometimes react inadequately to the aphasic's impairment.

Obviously, progress in the management of aphasia can only result from a better understanding of the aphasic patient's condition. As Biorn-Hansen (3) puts it, "by virtue of the complex interrelationship of emotions and the learning process, rehabilitation of the aphasic patient of necessity requires a comprehensive view of the total patient. This means recognizing many factors in the patient's life experience and evaluating the impact of these on the patient's ability to respond to training."

Valuable information on the aphasic patient's condition may be found in the accounts given by the disabled themselves. These accounts also raise a number of questions. The purpose of the present paper is to consider some of these questions together with their implications for the management of aphasia.

In the book called *Episode*, Eric Hodgins (8) reports that he was panic-striken when he found himself lying paralyzed and speechless on the floor of his flat. "I knew instantly what had happened to me: I had had a stroke", Hodgins relates. "Along with this knowledge, on a sort of parallel track, there rode the emotion of fear ... On the floor, something had happened to me ... and it was fearful—quite fearful" (p. 8).

Curiously enough, not every aphasic experiences the anguish which Hodgins was instantly overcome with. Stroke victims, in so far as they can remember their first post stroke days, often report that they were initially rather in-different. Scott Moss (12), who at 43 became aphasic following a cerebral artery thrombosis, notes that at the beginning of his illness "it was as if the stroke had benumbed any emotional investment in the future and I simply shrugged at the perception of my imminent demise". Helen Wulf too remained initially unconcerned: "I was totally unperturbed by the odd whatever-it-was that seemed to have control of me" (1973, p. 16). For some time after she had become aphasic and hemiplegic she lived in a sort of "care-free limbo" (p. 23).

Interestingly enough, in the novel *Les anneaux de Bicêtre* which depicts a businessman rendered suddenly aphasic by a stroke, Georges Simenon made the lack of concern about one's own handicap the main feature of his hero's state of mind during the first post-ictal days.

What can be the cause of this listlessness?

The initial indifference of many stroke patients to their incapacitation is probably the result of diaschisis. Though the insult destroys only part of the brain, its immediate effect is often to throw the whole cortical activity out of gear. This upsetting of the intellectual faculties prevents the patient from realizing the full scope of his impairment.

The possibility that the aphasic patient may be temporarily unconcerned about, or but partly aware of, his destitution should be born in mind especially if one insists (10, p. 25) that speech therapy be started as soon as possible after the onset of aphasia. A patient who is so shaken that he cannot fully appreciate his handicap, let alone be worried about it, is likely not to respond to therapy. On the other hand, if therapy begins a few weeks after the onset of aphasia, the first therapy sessions may coincide with the patient becoming aware of his deficits and their far-reaching consequences. Indeed, the therapy, because it sets the patient specific tasks, may cause the aphasic to suddenly realize the full scope of his verbal shortcomings, and this brutal discovery may affect his morale and self-confidence. It may even make him averse to pursuing therapy.

As regards the patient's buoyancy, another point to be heeded is the part which non-linguistic signs may come to play in his interaction with the environment. Helen Wulf points out how important her eyes had become at the beginning of her aphasia "to watch expressions on the faces of those around me ..., to look for gestures which can be wonderfully expressive ..., to search other eyes ..., to see smiles with their sunshine and healing" (p. 31).

Despite his word deafness a sensory aphasic can often be soothed and reassured by a loving voice or friendly looks. Wulf indicates that in the foggy bewilderment into which her aphasia had precipitated her, the only beacons were smiles and comforting intonations (p. 32). Indeed, the aphasic, because he finds words difficult to cope with, may attach undue significance to voice quality and to physiognomy, and this may lead to misunderstandings, and even to resentment.

Social intercourse with aphasics can also be complicated by a fluctuating word comprehension. When he was aphasic, Jacques Lordat, a professor at the faculty of medicine at Montpellier, France, was visited by two colleagues. As he failed to answer their questions as to how he felt and to follow the directions they gave him by way of test, the visitors thought that his verbal deafness was complete, and one of them remarked offhandedly that Lordat was done for. The patient eventually recovered, however, and he told his colleague that he had understood his disheartening prognosis and had laboured under it (2, p. 33).

Judgments as to comprehension difficulties in aphasics are often based on the patient's reactions to verbal commands. These reactions do not seem to form a really adequate criterion, however, since aphasics may find it difficult not only to understand words but also to turn words into actions. Albert, Yamadori, Gardner and Howes (1) had the opportunity to observe a patient who did not react to such written instructions as *Cough* or *Close your eyes*. However, specially devised reading tests revealed that he recognized the words.

The reason why some aphasics cannot translate words into actions may be that the left hemisphere is not only dominant for speech but also, as was suggested by Kimura and Archibald (9), for the execution of movements on request. Accordingly, when an aphasic fails to carry out an instruction, it should not be hastily concluded that he has not understood it. It may happen that he has grasped the order but cannot translate it into a motor sequence.

Moreover, it would appear that aphasics have less difficulty understanding messages they are interested in, or anxious to receive, than decoding questions or commands which are not related to their preoccupations. Lordat must have been eager to know what his colleagues thought of his condition and whether they deemed recovery possible. But trivial questions and test instructions must have left him indifferent.

It is as if in sensory aphasics the channel of speech reception had been narrowed by cerebral damage, so that understanding of information towards which the patient is biased is relatively preserved while other information is difficult to process. Such facilitating predisposition may to some extent also be observed in normals, at least under experimental conditions. Bruce (1958) had subjects repeat 5 tape-recorded sentences which were played back under admixture of noise. Every sentence was preceded by one of the five tag words *Sport, Food, Weather, Travel,* and *Health.* These words were played back without admixture of noise and were supposed to specify the contents of the sentence they introduced. The experiment was repeated five times, with a week's interval between two successive repetitions. Each time the order of presentation of the five sentences was different and each time each sentence was preceded by a different tag word. In one case, the tag word really fit the contents of the sentence. In the other four cases, it did not. The subjects did not know when the tag word actually corresponded to the contents of the sentence. Nonetheless, they repeated each sentence more faithfully when the tag word did correspond with the contents of the sentence. This means that because of the tag word the subjects were expectant of some definite contents; when the sentence had these contents, decoding was best.

In aphasia, too, expectancy often greatly facilitates comprehension. Therefore, in therapy and even more so in everyday life it seems desirable to prepare the patient for the reception of speech. Non-verbal cues can be used to bias him toward the verbal message one wants to communicate. Indeed, one should avoid addressing aphasics suddenly or asking them questions out of the blue. As one of the patients interviewed by Rolnick and Hoops (14) tried to put it: "After talking, then you can come as fast as you want to. But just sitting there, not having spoken to you or you to me ... all of a sudden you come out with some words, it takes time."

One should also refrain from talking to aphasics when they are engaged in an action. Wulf insists on her inability to deal with more than one thing at a time: "Everything must be done step by step", she notes, "one thing at a time, just one" (p. 19). Aphasics find it difficult to process speech while devoting part of their energy and attention to another activity. As Alonzo Hall (7), himself an aphasic, observes, even as simple an action as walking may require concentration on the part of the aphasic and hemiplegic patient, so that he cannot heed words when having to direct his steps over an uneven ground. In the same vein, Wulf remarks that "eating and carrying on an intelligent conversation is not always easy" (p. 119).

Within the confines of linguistic behaviour, twofold activity is difficult too. As Wulf points out, reading aloud often precludes comprehension (p. 119).

Wulf also remarks—with some sadness—that she no longer enjoys cartoons (p. 71). This is no isolated instance. Voinescu (in Lebrun and Hoops, 11, p. 80) found that aphasics are often unable to grasp the humour in picture stories. However, when the pictures forming a short comic are shown in disarray, these patients generally can rearrange them. It thus appears that they understand the events depicted in the comic but fail to see what is funny about them. In order to enjoy a cartoon one probably needs to perform a double intellectual task: to realize what the cartoon actually represents, and to appreciate in how far the portrayed event departs from common doings. The drawing in fact conveys a double meaning, and this is, it would seem, too much for the aphasic to cope with.

Semantic density also appears to lie at the root of the difficulty some aphasics have in dealing with disjunctive questions. A patient of Hildred Schuell's (15) indicated that he was at a loss when asked such a question as *Did you come by train or by bus?* "If the question had been 'Did you come by train?' it would have been easy to give a prompt and coherent reply", he explained. "But presenting an alternative places an obligation to both thought and speech."

A somewhat related difficulty was encountered by Wulf whenever she was handed a menu in a restaurant. She could not choose from the list of dishes (p. 123). A rather similar situation may obtain in alexia. Some alexics find it much more difficult to identify letters in words than letters presented in isolation (17).

Alternatives and equivalents may also be troublesome when the aphasic expresses himself. Butler (in Sies and Butler, 16), who became dysphasic following a motorcycle accident, reports that once he has formed an utterance, he finds it impossible to put together another sentence conveying the same thought. Consequently, when his interlocutor fails to understand him, Butler can only repeat his message: he cannot reword it. This often places him in an embarrassing situation which makes him shun conversation.

Another factor which may induce aphasics to avoid social contacts is fatigue. One year after the onset of aphasia Moss (12, p. 32) was again able to express himself but he found it exceedingly tiring to talk or to listen to a conversation for more than a few minutes on end.

However, extreme fatigability was not the only reason why Moss did not feel like socializing with friends and colleagues. He could not reconcile himself to his verbal shortcomings. "I haven't resigned myself yet to the fact that I am no longer as verbally fluent as I was earlier" he wrote. "This is a tremendous step for a person who throughout his lifetime could count on his ability to persuade others to his point of view and in effect sell his ideas through his ability to communicate" (p. 40). The French poet and essayist Valéry Larbaud must have felt the same after he became severely agrammatic. One day he came across some friends of his who inquired how he was. In dejection Valéry Larbaud answered *Déchu, déchu* i.e. degraded (5). In the same vein, Wulf notes that aphasia bereft her of her self-esteem (p. 36).

Aphasics not infrequently feel as if they were outcasts. The language impairment debars them from social intercourse and dooms them to solitude. Dr. Saloz, who for some time suffered from total motor aphasia, compared the aphasic's life with that of a victim immured in a tomb (13). Wulf laboured under "that awful feeling of being a prisoner within myself" (p. 51). And Hodgins calls the condition of the aphasic and hemiplegic patient a *living death* (p. 60).

When such despondency is present, it should be recognized and as far as possible remedied. Obviously, the patient's relatives must be involved. The speech therapist cannot hope to solve the problem without the collaboration of the patient's family. This sounds like a truism. All too often, however, speech therapists devote all their attention and energy to the treatment of the language disorder, thereby forgetting that aphasia is a familial problem.

These are some of the difficulties which aphasics are confronted with and which aphasia test batteries often fail to disclose, sophisticated as they may be. Those responsible for the management of aphasia cannot afford to ignore these difficulties, however, lest their efforts remain fruitless.

References

1. Albert, M., Yamadori, A., Gardner, H. & Howes, D.: Comprehension in alexia. Brain 96: 317, 1973.
2. Bayle, M.: Les fondateurs de la doctrine française de l'aphasie. Thesis. Bordeaux, 1939.
3. Biorn-Hansen, V.: Social and emotional aspects of aphasia. J Speech Hear Dis 22: 53, 1957.
4. Broca, P.: Du siège de la faculté du langage articulé. Bulletin de la Société d'Anthropologie 6: 377, 1865.
5. Constantin-Weyer, M.: Dans l'intimité de Valéry Larbaud. La Nouvelle Revue Française 5, 57: 421, 1957.
6. Griffith, V.: A Stroke in the Family. Penguin Books, Harmondsworth, 1970.
7. Hall, A.: Return from silence—A personal experience. J Speech Hear Dis 26: 174, 1961.
8. Hodgins, E.: Episode. Atheneum, New York, 1968.
9. Kimura, D. & Archibald, Y.: Motor functions of the left hemisphere. Brain 97: 337, 1974.
10. Knox, D.: Portrait of Aphasia. Wayne State University Press, Detroit, 1971.
11. Lebrun, Y. & Hoops, R.: Intelligence and Aphasia. Swets & Zeitlinger, Amsterdam, 1974.
12. Moss, S.: Recovery with Aphasia. University of Illinois Press, Urbana, 1972.
13. Naville, F.: Mémoires d'un médecin aphasique. Arch Psychol 17: 1, 1919.
14. Rolnick, M. & Hoops, H.: Aphasia as seen by the aphasic. J Speech Hear Dis 34: 48, 1969.
15. Schuell, H.: Paraphasia and paralexia. J Speech Hear Disord 25: 291, 1960.
16. Sies, L. & Butler, R.: A personal account of dysphasia. J Speech Hear Dis 28: 261, 1963.
17. Stachowiak, F. & Poeck, K.: Functional disconnection in pure alexia and color naming deficit demonstrated by facilitating methods. Brain and Language 3: 135, 1976.
18. Wulf, H.: Aphasia—My World Alone. Wayne Univ. Press, Detroit, 1973.

Glossolalia as a manifestation of Wernicke's aphasia: A comparison to glossolalia in schizophasia and in possession[1]

ANDRÉ ROCH LECOURS, LISA TRAVIS AND ELLEN OSBORN

Neologism and glossolalia

Two keywords of this paper are NEOLOGISM and GLOSSOLALIA. The first belonged, originally, to the vocabulary of philology, and the second to that of Christian religions. Both have nonetheless been used according to several interpretations attributed to them by students of various disciplines (including aphasiology and neurolinguistics). Each will be used here in line with a somewhat restrictive definition, formulated with the exclusive purpose of facilitating the description of certain deviant language behaviors. These two interdependent definitions will therefore bear no connotations other than taxonomical.

The word NEOLOGISM will designate individual spoken language segments uttered as if they were single words or locutions, and sharing three main characteristics. (*a*) They are phonologically articulated (1), that is, they can be described and transcribed as strings of conventionally pronounced phonemes. This excludes phonetically deviant segments such as those typical of the PHONETIC DISINTEGRATION commonly observed in BROCA'S APHASIA (2), or of other properly arthric disorders (3). (*b*) They are not to be found in the dictionaries of the language or languages the speaker masters or mastered through learning. This excludes lexically deviant segments such as the SEMANTIC PARAPHASIAS (e.g., 'hat'→"cover") commonly observed in certain forms of WERNICKE'S APHASIA (4), or the lapses by verbal substitution observed in ordinary language (5). (*c*) They do not individually represent transformations of precise conventional words or locutions that the listener can readily and confidently recognize on systematic formal clues. This excludes phonemically deviant segments such as the PHONEMIC PARAPHASIAS (e.g., 'policeman': 'agent de police': /aʒɑ̃dœpɔlis/→/aplaʒɑ̃dœplɔtis/) commonly observed in CONDUCTION APHASIA (6–8), or those—very much deliberate—of various entertainers. Apart from other types of deviant segments, the following excerpt from a conversation with a jargonaphasic patient comprises seven segments that would qualify as NEOLOGISMS according to the definition above: "*Tous les jours,*

[1] Work supported by grant MT-4210 of the *Conseil de la Recherche Médicale du Canada*.

elle venait à Paris pour /pale/ *dans les* /kɔsig/, *parce qu'elle prenait pour* ...
aussi pour entrer le ... *le palais—le palais normal, bien entendu—euh le*
/namytyʀ/, *la* /tɔktœʀ/ *et l'*/ɑ̃bœtjɛʀ/, *pour qu'elle sache tous ces* ... *ces choses,*
pour qu'elle sache à bien s'/ɛ̃skʀyme/, *à bien* ... *bien s'*/ɛ̃/ ... *bien s'*/ɛ̃kyme/."[1]

The word GLOSSOLALIA (1, 9–12) will designate any fluent euarthric spoken
discourse of some length that qualified—and circumspect—listeners will
perceive as entirely constituted of NEOLOGISMS or nearly so. Although both
words are commonly used to designate a single behavior (12), the notion of
GLOSSOLALIA thus differs from that of XENOGLOSSIA, the verbal behavior of
one who allegedly talks—when under the influence of a god, a devil or an
equivalent—one or several *bona fide* languages one has never learned. Thus
defined, glossolalic behavior can be observed to occcur in individuals of
several categories.

Glossolalic speakers

GLOSSOLALIA can occur as a very uncommon form of JARGONAPHASIA, observed mostly or only in the elderly (1). The clinical picture is then that of
severe and persistent WERNICKE'S APHASIA, with maximal impairment of
comprehension and of all but the arthric aspects of language production. In
such cases, GLOSSOLALIA is the direct result of acquired brain lesion. It
represents a residual behavior, i.e., it has become the only possible mode of
articulated speech production: it does not correspond to a deliberate choice.
The aphasic speaker with GLOSSOLALIA apparently remains unaware of the
anomalous nature of his utterances; whether or not he considers them to be the
embodiment of coherent thought remains an open question. As far as we
know, WERNICKE'S APHASIA is the only condition in which GLOSSOLALIA spontaneously occurs as a component of apparent dialogue. The following example
is excerpted from a "conversation" with such a patient (case W1):

[1] "/sɛ̃ dikte di tʀɔ̃ kɔ̃deʀe dʀikɔ̃dedeʀe digœʀe dis tis tilave klɔʀe œ le dø
tʀɔ̃ke ditibɛdœʀe disœ te kotegoʀe dil kɔ̃deteʀe/ /a wi dœ vilɛ̃bʀiʃ ʒe la
lɑ̃betɔʀi de dɛl lɑ̃tetɛʀœme di kategɔʀe/ /e œ e ɛlzekute ɛlmœpuʀimakɔ̃te
tɑ̃ tutse dœgʀedœgʀe dis gy lateʀe digeloteʀe/."

GLOSSOLALIA can also occur as a very uncommon form of SCHIZOPHASIA (1),
which has itself become—no doubt as a result of contemporary uses of chemo-
therapy—very uncommon among the schizophrenics. GLOSSOLALIA is then
episodical: it coexists with a capacity for standard language production. The
subject can define himself as the mere phonatory instrument of some mischiev-

---

[1] "Each day, she came to Paris in order to /pale/ in the /kɔsig/, because she took to ... also
to enter the ... the palace—the normal palace, of course—euh the /namytyʀ/, the /tɔktœʀ/
and the /ɑ̃bœtjɛʀ/, in order that she knows all of these ... these things, in order that she
knows at /ɛ̃skʀyme/ herself correctly, at ... at /ɛ̃/ ... at /ɛ̃kyme/ herself correctly."

ous will, for instance an enemy from a neighbouring village, country or planet. He is fully aware of the unconventional nature of his glossolalic utterances. A patient we have closely observed for several years claims that the phenomenon escapes the control of his own will but he is likely to glossolalize on demand. With regard to the messages behind his glossolalic utterances, this patient states (*a*) that they have precise meaning, (*b*) that formally identical utterances can have completely different meanings (maximal homophony is obviously the way he has found to corner us), (*c*) that he has no knowledge whatsoever of these meanings, and (*d*) that perhaps we might be able to decode and secretly profit by the alien message. The following example is excerpted from one of the interminable glossolalic monologues of this schizophasic patient (sample WF2):

[2] "/la manœRœpaRœ bRakal dœ Rœkɔ̃fjɔRezi ɛ̃tRøbeRogal dɔn yn bRibɛRgasjɔ̃ pinRomenal le baRjetegRal epineRopeRikal bRabal dœ Rœkɔ̃fjoRjasjɔ̃ pinRo-peRikal/ /yn bRibɛRgasjɔ̃ nemanaRœkaRœ bRabal dœ Rœkɔ̃fjoRjanis ɛ̃tRa-beRɔgad bRakal dœ Rœkɔ̃fjɔRezi ɛ̃tRøbɛRgal pineRomenal/."

Since the beginning of this century and more so in recent years, GLOSSOLALIA has once again become a rather common episodic behavior among believers in a strong and active Holy Ghost. The speaker typically defines himself as the willing although not deliberate phonatory instrument of the Ghost's ineffably benevolent will (11). He readily acknowledges the unconventional nature of his "inspired" utterances. He nonetheless believes these utterances to be meaningful in some archaic or contemporary human or angelic language; unless he is gifted with the charism of interpretation, he has no direct knowledge of the meaning of his own glossolalic productions. The following example is excerpted from a prayer (monologue) "spontaneously" uttered by a charismatic subject in the context of an *ad hoc* meeting (case CH4):

[3] "/putʃta jato amadea se atʃtu HORa o maRia ʃtuja talasul e maRja atunda asuja inʃtigoso jɛtʃteni/ /o maRja tuskundea deseu in dios kuna majʃte/ /o njanatʃe maRjana idonjaʃte koskena ɛ no njɔnɛskena/ /o niʃtɛne maRja tosɛ no no swɔʃtɛnei ɛ no ɛʃeRo swɔndinu udaʃse/."

Discussions with a well known and very clever exorcist have led us to suppose that persons possessed by the Devil are also prone to glossolalic episodes. It is said that the speaker is then the involuntary, perhaps reluctant, and purely executive tool of Mephistopheles. Here again, there would be precise meaning of which the speaker has no offhand knowledge. It is not clear to us if glosso-lalic speakers of this particular type are conscious or anosognosic of the unconventional nature of their utterances; at all events, they seem not to recol-lect having indulged in glossolalic behavior once appropriate procedures have lifted the spell. To this day and as far as we know, our corpus does not include samples of GLOSSOLALIA of demoniac origin.

Although this is not a rule and by far, there are children who, around age three or so, go through a period during which they occasionally engage in rather long stretches of euarthric and prosodically rich speech production that may sound very much neologistic.[1] As a rule, this is perceived by surrounding adults as selfaddressed monologue; or else, the child is apparently narrating, sometimes while turning the pages of a familiar illustrated story book, and he acts as if he considered his utterances meaningful and expected them to be understood.[2] Unless the listener is left with the impression that a strong proportion of the uttered segments are targetted on conventional words, this form of child behavior qualifies as GLOSSOLALIA according to our definition. Be that as it may, we have not yet found the energy necessary to follow one of the little fellows around, with an appropriate recording device, long enough to enrich our corpus with an acceptable sample of this type.

Somewhat to our surprise, we have found that a yet undetermined proportion of non-aphasic, non-schizophasic, non-believer, standard adult speakers, many of them agreeably histrionic, are perfectly capable, without any rehearsal nor previous glossolalic experience (active or passive), of long, fluent, convincing glossolalic monologues. This will occur in answer to instructions such as "try to talk as if talking in a language you do not know". Typically, such a subject will perform best or only if isolated in a quiet place and assuming a relaxed posture, with eyes closed; although very conscious and deliberate, she or he usually will insist on the importance of being "disconnected", whatever this means. These subjects do not assert that their glossolalic utterances correspond to precise sharable conventional messages. Most believe that a somewhat vague and fuzzy ideational mood favours glossolalic production, or might even be necessary for it. The following example is excerpted from the very first glossolalic monologue of a young lady who had no previous experience of GLOSSOLALIA and, indeed, who had never heard this word (case CR1):

[4] "/i evistimi tanto elevɛnte bɛste vanto elevɛsti bika anevɛnti mitistan elevɛnti liministaʀe inivindi me dastɔnte elekɛsti kue tikanto eliminimista batɛnto elevanta tɛstamɛnto alavinto e anvekemistan elividimistan elibidimistaj kede vete anto ivaj emindisti/."

We have found no adequate term to designate standard speakers capable of this type of production; we will refer to them as CR subjects ("CR" for creative).

Certain poets and professional entertainers have become famous for their glossolalic capacities. Theirs are of course deliberate and, in some uncon-

---

[1] A psychoanalyst friend recently wrote us the following about his then very talkative son: "Thomas' speech is at the same time incomprehensible and loaded with meaning. One wonders—and *he* obviously wonders—why this should not be attributed the status of a full-fledged language. Mimicry is there, and gestures as well, but the sounds are unexpected. But do not be mistaken. I understand perfectly well that he wants more yogurt, with maple syrup. Perhaps we should let him carry on ... and humanity would thereafter have been enriched with yet another language."

[2] Is this anosognosia?

	Wernicke	Schizophasic	Charismatic	Demoniac	Child	CR-Subject	Poet
Episodical behavior							
Ordinary people					+	+	+
Possessed people		+	+	+			
Residual behavior	+						
Documented brain lesion	+						
Label from official medicine	+	+					
Brain in maturation (13; 14)					+		
Anosognosia	+			?	?		
Deliberateness:							
Documented		+	+	?		+	+
Acknowledged		−	−	?		+	+
Meaningfulness claimed		+	+	+	+		+
Xenoglossia claimed		+	+	+			
Meaning believed inherent to sound							+

Fig. 1. Non linguistic characteristics of GLOSSOLALIA in speakers of various categories.

ventional way not unlike that of abstract painting, semantically purposeful productions. The listener may be left with an impression of improvisation but experience, rehearsals, as well as systematic use of paper and pencil are no doubt cornerstones of this particular mode of artistic expression. The following example is excerpted from the monologue of a (full time) poet and musician who was asked to "improvise" a stretch of GLOSSOLALIA, a performance with which he is very familiar (case P):

[5] "/œ̃ ʒuʀ le zalfal pʀiʀ lœ plupuf syʀ le byʀly bɛglyf/ /ɔʀ le byʀly bɛglyk
    ki kʀofaltɛ su lœ supʀœ̃tɛl aʀivɛʀ syʀ lœ bɔʀ dy slofɛl/ /lœ flofɛl sɔʀtɛ
    suvɑ̃ su lœ suflil mɛ kɔm lœ slɔ̃fɛl avɛ tuʒuʀ de bʀubuʃ de byʀly bɛglyk
    le nunu nana pʀyfi kɔ̃flɛ/."

As a skeleton of French syntax obviously guides the production in this sample, we hesitated before including it in our GLOSSOLALIA corpus.

Potential criteria for regrouping the above seven classes of glossolalic speakers in various manners can be summarized as shown in Figure 1.

Subjects and material

The GLOSSOLALIA material taken into consideration was obtained from two subjects with WERNICKE'S APHASIA (W1 and W2), one schizophrenic (SA, SD, SF1, SF2), five adepts of the Pentecostal faith (CH1 to CH5), two standard speakers (CR1 and CR2) and one poet (P). French was the mother tongue of all subjects; it was the only language fluently spoken in all but one case (W1). Unless otherwise specified, the first 2 000 phonemes of each sample were considered in the present study; when thought to be of interest, these were compared to various corpuses of aphasic and schizophasic language (native French speakers) and to various corpuses of idiomatic French.

The first aphasic patient (W1), a right-handed retired schoolteacher of *Auvergnat* stock, spoke both French and his provincial dialect fluently. His aphasia occurred when he was 79 years of age, as the result of radiologically circumscribed left posterior temporal softening (probably due to embolism). It began with suppression, soon and definitively to be replaced by fluent jargonaphasia. Graphism itself was normal, but written expression was reduced to slow repetitive production of a few letters and of two syllables that could be considered as grammatical words (*le* and *de*). All transposition behaviors[1] were severely impaired. Both oral and written comprehension were minimal. Anosognosia was apparently total. The sample considered in this paper was abstracted from a long and somewhat surrealistic "conversation" with this subject.

The second aphasic patient (W2), a right-handed widow whose native and only language was Québec French, suddenly became aphasic at the age of 76. Glossolalic jargon behavior followed a short period of suppression (about ten minutes long). Written expression was reduced to a few scrawls (produced reluctantly). All transposition behaviors were severely impaired. Both oral and written comprehension were minimal. Anosognosia was apparently total. There was a right visual field defect. A CT-scan, done approximately two weeks after onset of aphasia, showed a massive old infarct in the territory of the left posterior cerebral artery; if there was a more recent and smaller superficial temporal infarct on this side, it could not be distinguished among the radiological manifestations of very important cortical atrophy throughout the patient's brain. The glossolalic sample considered in this paper was in the form of dialogue (recorded conversation).

The schizophasic subject, a right-handed man, is now 47 years old. His formal schooling was brief; besides being a peacetime soldier for a while, he used to perform various odd jobs but has not been working for the past 15 years or so. He has been considered a schizophrenic of the paranoiac type since 1964. This diagnosis has been supported by the observation of several episodes comprising visual and auditory hallucinations as well as delirious behaviors.[2] For years, he has claimed to be the reluctant but forcefully subdued phonatory instrument of mischievous alien wills, perhaps of Martian origin, sending decodable but as yet undecoded messages through his mouth. On the whole, these are monotonous and repetitive (see example [2]), a fact the speaker readily acknowledges; they can be uttered in

---

[1] Repetition, reading aloud, writing from dictation, copy.
[2] CT-scans of this patient have shown his left lateral ventricle to be slightly larger than his right one. We were relieved when told that this can be a normal variant.

any of the three "languages" to which he refers as his French mode (*tempéra-ment français*; SF), his English mode (*tempérament anglais*; SA) and his funny mode (*tempérament drôle*; SD). Although he peremptorily states that his glossolalic discourse is in no way dependent on his will, this subject is likely to talk in any of his modes upon request (for hours if one is patient enough to listen). Samples of each mode will be considered in this study (SF1, SA, SD); an additional sample of a recently changing and allegedly enriched French mode (SF2) will also be included. All samples are in the form of monologues.

The five Pentecostal believers are three girls and two boys, all right-handed, in their late teens or early twenties, and all gifted with the "charism" of GLOSSOLALIA. All were recorded between ceremonies, in the context of a religious meeting. None was quite certain about her or his glossolalic discourse being xenoglossic but all claimed it might well be. In fact, they did not care much about this particular aspect of their charismatic utterances; all insisted, however, on the fact that GLOSSOLALIA is prayer, a monologue telling of love and praise. When asked to perform in front of a microphone, none objected but all explicitly doubted it could be done, arguing that it was up to the Holy Ghost, and not to the charismatic speaker, to decide when one should talk in tongues; none seemed surprised when each turned out to be capable of glossolalizing at a signal from the interviewer. The five samples thus obtained averaged 584 phonemes (CH1 to CH5; 442, 1240, 242, 532 and 463 phonemes respectively).

The CR subjects are right-handed young ladies. Both were 23 years old at the time of recording and neither had had previous experience of GLOSSOLALIA. They considered their glossolalic monologues (CR1 and CR2) to be essentially asemantic although potentially capable of conveying moods and feelings.

The poet is successful enough to earn a comfortable country life out of what he says, recites, sings and publishes. He asserts that phonemes bear intrinsic meanings and, therefore, that GLOSSOLALIA is, at a certain "language level", an effective semantic tool that can be domesticated. The glossolalic "improvisation" he recorded at our demand (P) is a monologue comprising 1,045 phonemes.

Our glossolalic corpus thus includes 14 samples. They were compared to samples of equal length (2,000 phonemes) from five control subjects: two ordinary speakers being interviewed on their daily work and life, one non glossolalic patient with SCHIZOPHASIA and one with JARGONAPHASIA [numerous deviations of all types in both cases (1, 4)] and one patient with CONDUCTION APHASIA [fluent discourse comprising numerous phonemic deviations (4)]. Massive data on the incidence of phonemes in spoken French were also used for reference; they were Santerre's for Québec (15) and Lafon's for France (16).

Suprasegmental aspects

When compared to normals, the jargonaphasic and schizophasic controls displayed no gross differences as far as prosody is concerned. This was also found to be the case of the W and P samples in our glossolalic corpus. This cannot be said of the S, CH and CR samples, where several aspects of prosody deserve being mentioned, namely general melody, speed of elocution, regional accent and tonic accent.

General melody

Although general melody differs from one sample to another, even perhaps from one category of glossolalic speakers to another, there seems to exist a major melodical investment[1] in all but the aphasic subjects and the poet. In both the French and the English modes, the melody of the S samples is monotonous and it rather closely mimics the tone which is familiar to any listener of short-waves ideological transmissions, whether from Radio Free Europe, the Voice of America or Radio Tirana. It should therefore be pointed out that the patient once told us how elated he felt when listening, for hours in a row, to foreign broadcasting he could not understand. All we can say of the melody in sample SD is that it strikes us as going far astray from that in ordinary language. In sample CH2, the general melody is clearly that of forceful imprecation; in the four other CH samples, it is clearly that of fervent prayer. Both types of melodic investment have been observed by students of charismatic glossolalia (21, 22). In the CR samples, general melody is best described as recitative and/or theatrical. In this respect, CR subjects will occasionally comment on their greater deliberateness in prosodical choices as compared to phonological ones.

Speed of elocution

Elocution speed also varies widely from one sample to another. Grossly, there are those who take about 15 seconds to utter 100 phonemes and convey an impression of ordinary speed of elocution (apart from the normal controls, this includes the CR and P subjects), those who convey an impression of very fast declamation, in which uttering 100 phonemes can take as little as 7 seconds (this includes the S subject in all modes and subject CH2, that is, the one with the imprecatory melody), and finally the slow talkers, who take between 25 and 45 seconds to utter 100 phonemes (this includes the W subjects and the four CH subjects with the prayer-like melody).

---

[1] It is of interest, incidentally, that one of the aphasics (W1), the schizophasic and two of the charismatics actually engaged in glossolalic songs while being recorded.

Regional accent

The regional accent of Québécois French, the characteristics of which are easily perceived and described, is very much attenuated in the four S samples and it completely disappears in the CH and CR samples. Nothing of the sort occurs in the W and P samples.

Tonic accent

Much to our surprise, at least initially, we found that the expected regular French oxytone was partially or totally replaced by a paroxytone in all CH and CR samples, as well as in the SA and SD samples. Let us therefore point out that, although unilingual, the S, CH and CR subjects had all been previously prone to attentive listening of foreign languages such as Italian, Spanish, Greek and English. It is also noteworthy that samples F1 and F2 from the schizophasic subject (French *tempérament*), as well as the W and P samples remained oxytone throughout.

Segmental aspects

Listeners of glossolalic utterances nearly always remain with the very definite impression that they have heard a multiarticulated discourse, that is, a discourse composed of simpler units being combined into progressively more complex ones (17): a discourse comprising units assimilable to phonemes, syllables, words (sometimes with several morphemic components), and sentences. An it-sounds-like reaction is common: "It sounds like Greek, Hebrew, Chinese" and so forth.

Provided a set of rules, phonemic and syllabic segmentation is no more a source of difficulty than if one was dealing with natural tongues one does not know. On the whole, segmentation in sentence-like entities is not a problem either, in view of relatively clear prosodical clues and longer pauses. On the other hand, and but for a certain proportion of strongly word-like segments, it is often difficult or impossible to reach common agreement of several listeners on word-like level segmentation (a fact that should be kept in mind when considering the examples quoted above). This proportion of strongly word-like segments varies widely from one sample to another, depending mostly on pauses and melodical clues, on recurrence of identical or similar strings and their tonic accent, on amount of affix-like entities, and on greater or lesser occurrence of real dictionary words (especially of those belonging to grammatical inventories: for instance, it is easy to recognize neologistic word-like segments in 'The /gilub/ has /pɔstigaʀtœd/ the /blɛtʃ/', a fictitious example). Although apparently a futile venture in certain cases, the pertinency of segmentation in word-like entities is thus somewhat substantiated in others;

seeking the collaboration of the glossolalic speaker (if not an aphasic) can be useful—and perhaps misleading—in this respect, as well as considering eventual written productions (GLOSSOGRAPHIA).

Phonemic frequencies

In most of our samples, all of the uttered sounds are assimilable to phonemes of the French inventory; samples SD, CH2, CH5 and CR2 are also French-like in this respect but comprise a few foreign-sounding segments (less than 1 %), most of which are assimilable to English /r/, /l/ and /H/ (which is hardly an anomaly in Québécois French). All samples are thus essentially native language as far as phonemic choices are concerned.

As can easily be seen perusing through *Table I*, the frequency of individual phonemes is often different, sometimes grossly so, from that in standard conversational French. The outstanding facts are (*a*) marked increase or (*b*) absence[1] or near absence of some of the most frequent phonemes in the idiom, and (*c*) marked increase of some of the less frequent phonemes in the idiom (see, for instance, increase of /d/ in W1, absence of /t/ and decrease of /R/ in SA, increase of /ʃ/ in CH1, etc.). This particular pattern of phonemic distribution was observed in all of the glossolalic samples but in none of the controls (whether the latter were normal, jargonaphasic or schizophasic speakers). Therefore, we tend to consider it as characteristic.

Several questions arise from closer examination of the data in *Table I*. Why, for instance, should different glossolalic speakers share predilection phonemes, especially if these are somewhat infrequent in the mother tongue, e.g., why should the two W subjects, the S subject (in all four of his *tempéraments*), one of the CR subjects and the poet share a very definite predilection for /b/, whereas all five of the CH subjects either underemploy this particular phoneme or altogether abandon it. Well, we cannot answer this question (no psycho-analytic formation). On the other hand, this increase of /b/ reflects, in both W cases, a more generalized increase of the voiced stops (/b/, /d/ and /g/ in W1; /b/ and /g/ in W2). Given known data on the fragility of voiced consonants in the aphasic transformations of French and English speaking subjects (18 to 20), could not one consider this as indirect evidence that glossolalic jargonaphasia is not targetted, i.e., that it does not represent maximal transformation of precise words and sentences?

Phonemic combinations

Just as phoneme-like segments in our glossolalic samples are permitted given the French phonemic inventory, so are their modes of combination permitted

---

[1] The most striking fact we have observed so far in this respect is the total absence of inter-dentals and diphthongs in the long glossolalic productions of three (charismatic) native speakers of English, recorded in London by Paolo Fabbri and Sylvano Fua (Centro Internazionale di Semiotica e Linguistica, Urbino, and R.A.I., Rome).

Table I. *Santerre's data on the frequency of phonemes in Québec French (15) and* Frequency of phonemes in 14 glossolalic samples and 5 control samples. Q: native speakers of Québec about their daily work and life. S control is excerpted from a sample of archetypical schizophasia case of conduction aphasia (4). Samples W are from patients with glossolalic jargonaphasia, sample from ordinary speakers, and sample P from a poet.

	Santerre (15)	Lafon (16)	Q control	F control	Sample W1 (F)	Sample W2 (Q)	Sample SA (Q)	Sample SD (Q)	Sample SF1 (Q)	Sample SF2 (Q)
/p/	4.4	4.3	4.1	3.9	1.6	5.6	2	2.5	1.7	2.4
/b/	1.3	1.2	0.7	1.6	3.2	3.1	8.6	3.8	6.9	6.8
/m/	3.4	3.4	4.2	4.5	3.4	5.2	4.4	2.9	1.4	1.5
/t/	5	4.5	5.1	5.1	4.5	3.7	0	0.5	3.2	2.9
/d/	3.7	3.5	5.3	3.1	10.7	2	0.1	0.6	3.4	2.6
/n/	2.5	2.8	2.4	1.8	0.4	1.4	2	0.8	4.8	5
/k/	3.6	4.5	3.3	4	3.4	3.1	7.7	13.5	5.6	3.7
/g/	0.5	0.3	0.4	0.3	3.3	1.4	2.8	1.4	1.8	2.8
/ɲ/	0.1	0.1	0.1	0.2	0	0	0.1	0	0	0.1
/f/	1.3	1.3	2.2	1.4	0.3	0.5	0	0.5	1.8	1.4
/v/	2.3	2.4	2.2	2.3	0.8	2.6	0	0.4	0.7	0.4
/s/	5.9	5.8	6.3	6.6	1	6	4.5	2.8	3.1	2.3
/z/	1.4	0.6	1	1.7	0.2	2.5	4.7	1.2	0.8	0.8
/ʃ/	0.6	0.5	0.2	0.7	0.5	1.1	0	0.3	0.2	0
/ʒ/	2.2	1.7	3.2	2.2	0.4	2.4	0	0.1	0.1	0.2
/l/	6.5	6.8	4.7	5.9	6.8	2.4	0.2	17.4	5.4	6.8
/ʀ/	6.4	6.9	7.1	7.4	9.3	3.4	19.2	1.8	13.9	14.4
/ʜ/	0	0	0	0	0	0	0	0.1	0	0
/j/	2.1	1	2.1	1.5	0.2	3.4	4.4	1.1	4.2	4.5
/w/	1.6	0.9	1.6	1.1	0.4	1.8	0	0.3	0.4	0.1
/ɥ/	1.1	0.7	0.2	0.7	0.1	0.3	0	0	0	0
/i/	5.4	5.6	4.1	6.2	6.5	3.9	2.7	11.4	4.2	5.5
/y/	1.8	2	2.3	1.2	2.7	1.2	0	0.5	0.8	0.3
/u/	2	2.7	1.2	1.9	1	0.9	3.5	5	0.3	0.1
/e/	6.1	6.5	6.7	6.6	13.4	8.3	0.3	3.2	4.7	8.2
/ø/	0.5	0.6	0.9	1	0.8	1	0	0	0.4	1.6
/o/	1.3	1.7	0.5	1.1	3.2	0.5	6.1	0.5	0.7	1.3
/ɛ/	5.3	5.3	4.4	5.8	4.2	3.6	10.1	1	1.3	1.2
/œ/	2.9	5.2	3.9	1.6	6.9	11.7	3.8	5.3	4	3.2
/ə/	1.4	1.5	1.8	1.8	1.2	2.5	0	0.2	4.9	3.4
/a/	6.6	8.1	10.1	8.2	2.4	4.9	12.3	6.4	10.8	10.9
/ɑ/	3.6	0.2	0.8	0.2	0.1	5.1	1.2	15	2.6	2
/ɛ̃/	1.2	1.4	1.2	1.2	1.1	2.2	0	0.1	2.1	1.4
/œ̃/	0.4	0.5	0.7	0.8	0.1	0.5	0	0	0.1	0
/ɑ̃/	3.3	3.3	4	3.9	2.5	0.8	0	0	1.5	0.4
/ɔ̃/	2.2	2	1	2.5	3.4	1	0	0	2.7	2.8

Lafon's data on the frequency of phonemes in France French (16)

French. F: native speaker of France French. Q and F controls are from ordinary speakers telling (1), J control from an archetypical case of neologistic jargon (4), and C control from an archetypical S from a patient with glossolalic schizophasia, samples CH from Pentecostal believers, samples CR

Sample CH1 (Q)	Sample CH2 (Q)	Sample CH3 (Q)	Sample CH4 (Q)	Sample CH5 (Q)	Sample CR1 (Q)	Sample CR2 (Q)	Sample P (Q)	S control (F)	J control (F)	C control (F)
0.7	0	0	0.2	2.4	0.1	2.2	4.3	3.9	3	2.6
0	0.1	0	0	0	1	3.5	4.4	0.9	1.4	1.2
6.3	7.3	5.4	2.6	1.5	5.7	6.2	1.6	3.5	4.2	3
5	0.1	0	8.5	6.9	12.2	10.6	3.7	5.5	6	6.4
0.9	0.3	0	5.1	1.5	1.8	0.7	3.5	4.1	3.6	5.1
0.2	6.9	21.9	10.7	7.5	10.7	0.5	1.8	2.8	2.7	1.5
6.6	16	10	2.2	5.2	2.6	6.5	3.9	5.5	4.1	3.8
0	0.5	0	0.6	0.2	0.1	0.4	0.8	0.3	0.1	0.8
0	0	0	0.2	0.2	0.1	0.5	0.2	0.1	0	0
0	0	0	0	0.2	0.1	0.3	3.6	1.4	0.9	2
0	0	0	0	0	4.6	0.1	2.2	2.5	1.4	2.5
3.2	0	0.4	5.6	5.6	3.3	0.4	4.4	5.8	6.5	5.4
0	0.1	0	0.2	0	0	0.1	0.5	1.3	1.1	1.6
8.4	4.4	4.1	5.3	1.7	0.9	2.9	1.3	0.3	0.7	0.7
0	0	0	0	0	0	0	0.2	0.4	3.2	3.8
5.6	7.3	0	1.7	3.2	4.5	6.2	11.2	7	6.3	5.2
7.9	6.5	0	2.6	6.9	2.1	3.4	10	6.8	6.3	5.8
0	0.4	0	0.2	0.9	0	0	0	0.1	0	0
1.6	3	0.8	6.8	9.3	2.8	5.4	1.2	1.8	1.4	1.5
0	1.3	7	0.6	0.9	0.1	1.5	0.3	0.9	2	1.2
0	0	0	0	0	0.1	0	0	0.1	0.9	0.3
15.4	2.7	11.6	6	9.1	11.7	9.9	5.8	5.5	4.7	3.1
0	1.9	0	0	0	0.2	0.3	4.5	3.4	1.1	1.6
2.3	4.4	0	4.7	0.6	0.3	13.6	5	2.1	2.8	2.3
4.7	4.8	3.7	7.3	11.7	8.2	1.2	5.1	4.9	4.9	7.7
0	0	0.5	0	0	0.1	0.2	0.2	0.6	0.2	0.2
7	6.3	4.9	7.5	3.9	3.6	2.3	2	1.6	0.9	1.8
0	2.9	0	4.3	2.2	4	0.8	3.8	4.9	6.5	6.1
0	0.2	0	0.2	1.1	3	0.1	1.7	5	4.9	5.6
0	5.3	0	1.9	1.9	1.2	1.2	1.5	2.4	2	2.1
24.2	6.6	30.2	15	15	6.6	12.6	4.2	8.6	8.2	9.3
0	10.6	0	0	0.4	3.6	6	1.2	0.1	0.2	0.1
0	0	0	0	0	0	0	1.6	1	1.5	0.8
0	0	0	0	0	0	0	0.6	0.7	0.3	0.1
0	0.1	0	0	0	0.1	0.7	0.6	2.6	4.4	3
0	0.1	0	0	0	0	0.5	2	1.6	1.3	1.8

given the French phonological system.[1] Glossolalic utterances are therefore phonologically rule-governed[2] (1). Here again, however, enslavement to mother tongue stops at this point in all samples. In other words, combinations which are frequent in the mother tongue can be utterly neglected, and infrequent ones can become predilection linkages.[3] Moreover, only a small proportion of possible combinations are actualized in any given sample.

On the whole, these segmental characteristics of glossolalic production are more obvious in the S, CH and CR samples than in the W and P samples. This is true of both the pattern of phonemic frequencies and the pattern of phonemic combinations.

Now, if one chooses consonant clusters as a parameter of phonological complexity, further characterization of our material emerges. As opposed to one of the normative samples, which comprises 21.3% of phonemes within consonantic clusters (/R/ and /l/ included), the P sample exemplifies increased complexity (34.2%) and the W samples exemplify decreased complexity (10.8% in W1 and 8.4% in W2). Both phenomena are immediately perceptible to the listener's ear. Other samples range from the simplest to the most complex; when the latter occurs, nonetheless, clusters remain qualitatively few (i.e., the same clusters recur over and over again).

Families of word-like segments

Within any glossolalic sample of some length, one can identify inventories of word-like segments which bear to one another formal relationships that are not unlike those between PHONEMIC PARAPHASIAS and corresponding target words (6). Rules governing such relationships, in the glossolalic material, are usually rather simple. In the following example, excerpted from sample W1, several vocalic permutations are possible in all but the last syllable, and a few consonantal permutations are possible in the third syllable, less often in the second one:

[6] /kategɔʀe/	/kɔ̃tegœʀe/
/kotegoʀe/	/kotedœʀe/
/kɑ̃tegoʀe/	/kɔ̃tedœʀe/
/kɑ̃tɛgœʀe/	/kɔ̃tebœʀe/
/kɔ̃tɛgɔʀe/	/kɔ̃deteʀe/ etc.

---

[1] Although certain phonemic combinations that are probably acceptable only at word boundaries in standard French may occur within entities that most listeners perceive as word-like.

[2] *Suppression* would, in our opinion, be the clinical manifestation of severe dysfunction of or damage to—whatever its localization or specificity—the neuronal net subtending, through learning, phonologically rule-governed oral language production.

[3] When associated to a few unexpected phonemic choices and/or to change in tonic accent (Cf. *supra*), this contributes to giving glossolalic utterances a superficial foreign shade which, in turn, may account for many a claim to xenoglossic competence (12).

In [7], an example excerpted from sample SA, all consonants are stable and vowel permutations are possible in all syllables. If one considers this particular inventory as a whole, one frequently has the impression of anterograde or retrograde assimilations or dissimilations:

[7] /kɛʀœkuʀu/   /kɛʀɛkuʀu/
   /kɛʀœkoʀo/   /kɛʀɛkoʀo/
   /kɛʀœkoʀu/   /kɛʀakuʀu/
   /kɛʀokoʀu/   /kɛʀakoʀo/
   /kɛʀokoʀo/   /kaʀakuʀu/
   /kɛʀəkoʀo/   /kaʀœkuʀu/
   /kɛʀəkəʀu/   /kaʀœkoʀo/ etc.

Rules are somewhat more complex in [8], an example excerpted from sample CH2. They allow various permutations on all vowels and second consonant, reciprocal metathesis on first and second consonant, and expansion on first and third consonant as well as second vowel:

[8] /m ana kala/   /m əna ʃkolo/
   /m ana kolo/   /mw ana ʃkolo/
   /m ono kolo/   /mw anai ʃkolo/
   /m ona kale/   /m ala ʃkolo/
   /m ala kala/   /m ala ʃkəlu/
   /m ana ʃkala/   /m aja ʃkəle/
   /m ono ʃkolo/   /m ana ʃkole/
   /m ana ʃkolo/   /m əna ʃkole/
   /n ama ʃkolo/   /m ono ʃkyli/ etc.

These inventories are usually established within relatively short stretches of glossolalic production. In our opinion, therefore, and contrary to charismatic leader Laurentin's contention (12), this very phenomenon suffices to distinguish glossolalic utterances from ordinary utterances in any natural language.

Derivation in word-like segments

In all of our samples, although more so in the non aphasic ones, we have observed the occurrence of sets of word-like segments in which derivation rules of a sort seemed to have been applied. In sample W1, for instance, the patient used the following word-like segments: [9] /mɛtʀ/, /ade-mɛtʀ/, /dig-ɛtʀo-mɛtʀ/, /dik-eli-mɛtʀ/, /dik-ãte-dœʀe/, /gyl-ãte-dœʀe/, /gyl-ɔ̃te/, etc. In sample CH2, one finds [10] /adɛ-ʃte/, /maj-ʃte/, /sni-ʃte/, /ido-nja-ʃte/, /jɛt-ʃte-ni/, /ni-ʃte-ne/, etc. In sample CR1, one finds [11] /anto/, /el-anto/, /el-am-anto/, /el-ev-anto/, /el-ev-ɛsti/, /in-im-anto/, etc. One of the most complex set we have observed is from sample SF1:

[12] /baʀjeteʀezi/:   /   baʀ jeteʀ ezi/
     /ʀœkɔ̃fəʀjaneʀezi/:   /ʀœ kɔ̃   fəʀ janeʀezi/
     /ʀœkɔ̃fjəʀezi/:   /ʀœ kɔ̃   fjəʀ   ezi/
     /ʀœkɔ̃fjəʀani/:   /ʀœ kɔ̃   fjəʀ   ani/
     /ʀœkɔ̃fjəʀanis/:   /ʀœ kɔ̃   fjəʀ   anis/
     /ʀœkɔ̃fjəʀasjɔ̃/:   /ʀœ kɔ̃   fjəʀ   asjɔ̃/
     /kɔ̃stʀasjɔ̃/:   /   kɔ̃   stʀ   asjɔ̃/
     /kɔ̃tʀavizeʀjasjɔ̃/:   /   kɔ̃tʀa vizeʀj   asjɔ̃/
     /beʀegasjɔ̃/:   /   beʀeg   asjɔ̃/
     /bʀibɛʀgasjɔ̃/:   /   bʀibɛʀg   asjɔ̃/
     /bʀibɛʀgasjəne/:   /   bʀibɛʀg   asjə ne/
     /bʀibɛʀgasjənis/:   /   bʀibɛʀg   asjə nis/
     /bʀibɛʀgal/:   /   bʀibɛʀg   al/
     /bʀabal/:   /   bʀab   al/
     /ɛ̃tʀabeʀəgal/:   /   ɛ̃tʀa beʀəg   al/
     /epinəʀmenal/:   /   epi   nəʀmen   al/
     /binəʀmenal/:   /   bi   nəʀmen   al/
     /mɑ̃tʀalite/:   /   mɑ̃tʀ   al   ite/ etc.

Sentence-like segments

It should be clear, by now, that all of our glossolalic samples comprise predilection segments of various levels of complexity.[1] This phenomenon—which one might wish to call *perseveration* although this is probably too pervasive a term to be useful in the present context—can involve phonemes (*Table I*), syllables and other phonemic combinations, morpheme-like and word-like segments, even phrase-like and sentence-like segments in certain cases (S, CH and C samples). When the latter occurs, the listener may be left with the impression of an endless repetition of the same sentence-like entity. This is only partially substantiated by attentive listening and transcription. Even in caricatural cases, word-like segments indeed behave, within predilection sentence-like contexts, in the same manner phonemes behave within predilection word-like contexts (Cf. supra, examples [6] to [8]), that is, rule-governed variations are permitted within certain limits. Let us consider sample SA, by far the most repetitive in our corpus, in order to illustrate this point. This sample comprises 13 different word-like segments. Most of these, as illustrated in example [7], can have variants. In their most frequent forms, these word-like segments are the following:

1 = /azumba/   5 = /paʀa/
2 = /bɛʀgɛs/   6 = /bʀazjɛ mnɛʀgɛs/
3 = /koʀo/   7 = /aʀakaska ʀœkaʀœ/
3' = /keʀœkoʀu/   8 = /misi/
4 = /bʀubjɛʀ/   8' = /mizœpʀiz/.

[1] These are sometimes distributed more or less evenly throughout the sample, and sometimes they are relatively restricted to certain parts of it.

As shown in 6, 7 and 8' above, some of these word-like segments are inseparable or nearly so. Three other groupings are frequent:

a $= (3$ or $3' + 4)$
A $= (5 + 6 + a)$
B $= (8' + 7 + 6 + a)$.

The structures of all of the sentence-like entities in sample SA can thus be summarized as follows:

$$S = {\ }+1\pm2+a+ \begin{vmatrix} A \\ \text{or:} \\ B \end{vmatrix} \pm A + \begin{vmatrix} 8 \\ \text{or:} \\ (B+8) \\ \text{or:} \\ (B+B+8) \\ \text{or:} \\ (B-4) \end{vmatrix},$$

where $+$ precedes compulsory and $\pm$ facultative components. For instance:

[13] /azumba | bɛʀgɛs | koʀo bʀubjɛʀ | paʀa bʀazja mnɛʀgɛs keʀɔkoʀo bʀubjɛʀ | mizœ pʀiz aʀakaska ʀœkaʀœ bʀazjɛ mnɛʀgɛs keʀakoʀo/.

[14] /azumba | bɛʀgɛs | koʀo bʀubjɛʀ | paʀa bʀazjɛ mnɛʀgɛs keʀakoʀo buʀbjɛʀ | mizœ pʀiz aʀakaska ʀœkaʀœ bʀazja mnɛʀgɛs keʀakoʀo bʀubjɛʀ | misi/.

[15] /azaʀœ | koʀo bʀobjɛʀ | paʀa bʀasja mnɛʀgɛs kɛʀœkoʀo bʀobjɛʀ | miza pʀiz aʀakaska ʀakaʀœm bʀasja mnɛʀgɛs kɛʀokoʀo bʀobjɛʀ | miza pʀiz aʀakaska ʀakaʀa bʀazja mnɛʀgɛs keʀokoʀu bʀɔbjɛʀ | mesi/.

[16] /azaʀa | kuʀu bʀubjɛʀ | paʀa bʀasja minɛʀgɛs kɛʀœkuʀu bʀubjɛʀ | mizœ pʀiz aʀakaska ʀœkaʀœ bʀasja minɛʀgɛs kaʀœkuʀu bʀubjɛʀ mizœ pʀiz aʀakaska ʀakaʀa bʀazja minɛʀgɛs kɛʀokoʀu bʀubjɛʀ | mesi/.

Summary and conclusion

As we have defined it, GLOSSOLALIA can occur in subjects of different categories. We have personally observed it in aphasic and schizophasic subjects, as well as in Pentecostal believers (CH subjects) and ordinary speakers (CR subjects). In this study, we have considered both suprasegmental and segmental aspects of GLOSSOLALIA.

A major melodic investment was observed in all but three samples (W1, W2 and P). Regional accent was preserved in the aphasics but attenuated or abandoned in the S, CH and CR subjects who, at times, also replaced the expected Frenchlike oxytone for a paroxytone. In our opinion, these prosodic modifications in the S, CH and CR samples could be accounted for by informal exposure, the source of which might have been radio listening and similar activities.

Segmental aspects of glossolalic behavior were also taken as being related to exposure (if only because it could hardly be otherwise). Phonetic realization proper was conventional in all samples, i.e., we did not observe any dysarthric component to GLOSSOLALIA. Phonemic choices and combinations were also rule-governed: they corresponded, entirely or quasi entirely, to choices and combinations permitted in French, the mother tongue of all of our subjects. The same was true of the few morphemic choices and combinations detected in each sample (see examples [9] to [12]). In some of the S, CH and CR samples, minor and very restricted loans from foreign languages were also possible at both phonological and morphological levels, a fact we have also observed in native speakers of Italian and English indulging in GLOSSOLALIA. This can no doubt be accounted for by exposure to foreign languages, however limited. All samples were shown to comprise inventories of word-like units bearing to one another structural relationships reminiscent of those between PHONEMIC PARAPHASIAS and corresponding target words (see examples [6] to [8]): as far as we know, this does not occur—at least to this extent—in natural languages. Preferential use of segments of various levels of complexity (predilection units: phonemes, phonemic associations, word-like segments, etc.) was found in all samples. This phenomenon reached the sentence level in certain cases, therefore leaving the listener with an impression of endless repetition. Only in part was this impression substantiated: word-like segments were observed to behave, within sentence-like segments, in the same manner phonemes did within word-like segments, i.e., rule-governed variations regularly occurred (see examples [6] to [8] and [13] to [16]).

In the elderlies, GLOSSOLALIA is sometimes observed as a manifestation of severe WERNICKE'S APHASIA. This is the only condition in which it results from brain lesion and represents a residual behavior. This is also the only condition in which GLOSSOLALIA spontaneously occurs as a component of apparent dialogue. In spite of assertions to the contrary by S and CH subjects, as well as by students of schizophasic and charismatic GLOSSOLALIA (12, 23), the initiation of glossolalic behavior was observed to be deliberate in all of our subjects without brain lesions, including the schizophasic and all five charismatics; thus, lack of deliberateness also proved to be a distinctive characteristic of the aphasics among the glossolalic speakers we have recorded. Another distinctive characteristic was anosognosia, which was present in both W subjects but in none of the others.

Other differences were noted between the two W patients and the other glossolalics. For instance, elocution speed was found to be relatively diminished in the two aphasics while it could be exaggerated, sometimes verging on virtuosity, in some of the non aphasics. Likewise, the complexity of glossolalic utterances, as judged on consonant clusters, was less than that of mother tongue in the two W samples and greater than that of mother tongue in the P sample, which makes sense. On the whole, however, the discourse of both W patients shared structural features with that of non aphasic glossolalic speakers somewhat more than with that of other aphasics, including those with neologistic jargon (see Table I, J control and C control).[1] Two of these features deserve explicit mention: on the one hand, a particular pattern of phonemic frequencies and combinations, which emerges when comparison is made to mother tongue (Table I); on the other hand, the constitution of characteristic inventories of formally related word-like segments (see examples [6] to [8]). Moreover, there is indirect evidence that glossolalic jargonaphasia, like GLOSSOLALIA in non aphasic speakers but unlike other varieties of JARGONAPHASIA (4), is not a targeted production, i.e., does not represent the phonemic transformation of conventional words and sentences, i.e., is asemantic or nearly so.

Whether or not GLOSSOLALIA is being observed in subjects with brain lesions, and whether or not one considers that glossolalic speakers with and without brain lesions share more than superficial similarity in phonatory behavior, the very existence of GLOSSOLALIA leads to the formulation of several questions that are of fundamental interest from the neurological point of view. None of these questions can, for the time being, be given a satisfactory answer. We do not know, for instance, which are the brain structures that subserve glossolalic behavior in the subject without brain lesion; we do not know if these structures are lateralized and, if so, on which side (in this respect, we are struck by the kinship between glossolalic behavior and musical improvisation); and we do not know if the activities of certain brain structures need be inhibited for glossolalic behavior to take place. We also do not know which brain lesions are likely to reduce one's linguistic capacities to glossolalic behavior (in this respect, we are struck by the fact that glossolalic jargonaphasia occurs only in the elderly); and we do not know if these lesions are unilateral—left?—or bilateral, nor if they have to spare certain cortical or subcortical structures for the glossolalic release to actualize. In relation to this problem, we are not ready to forget this patient, observed over a period of nine years (24), who was capable of fluent, euarthric but completely ineffective discourse in spite of verified lesions destroying not only Wernicke's area proper, but also the central operculum, the insula and Heschl's zone in the left hemisphere, as well as Broca's area and its homologue in the right hemisphere.

References

1. Lecours, A. R. & Vanier-Clément, M.: Schizophasia and jargonaphasia: A comparative description with comments on Chaika's and Fromkin's respective looks at 'schizophrenic' language. Brain and Language 3: 516, 1976.
2. Alajouanine, Th., Ombredane, A. & Durand, M.: Le syndrome de désintégration phonétique dans l'aphasie. Masson, Paris, 1939.

[1] The same could be said of our S samples when comparison is made to other glossolalic samples as opposed to samples of schizophasic language without glossolalia (see Table I, S control).

3. Darley, F. L., Aronson, A. E. & Brown, J. R.: Differential diagnostic patterns of dysarthria. J Speech Hear Res 12: 246, 1969.
4. Lecours, A. R. & Rouillon, F.: Neurolinguistic analysis of jargonaphasia and jargonagraphia. In: H. Whitaker & H. Whitaker (eds.), Studies in Neurolinguistics, vol. II, p. 95. Academic Press, New York, 1976.
5. Fromkin, V. A.: Speech Errors as Linguistic Evidence. Mouton, the Hague, 1973.
6. Lecours, A. R. & Lhermitte, F.: Phonemic paraphasias: Linguistic structures and tentative hypotheses. Cortex 5: 192, 1969.
7. Geschwind, N.: Aphasia. New Engl J Med 284: 654, 1971.
8. Buckingham, H. W. & Kertesz, A.: Neurolinguistics 3: Neologistic Jargon. Swets and Zeitlinger, Amsterdam, 1976.
9. Cénac, M.: De certains langages créés par les aliénés: contribution à l'étude des glossolalies. Thèse, Faculté de Médecine, Paris, 1925.
10. Bobon, J.: Introduction historique à l'étude des néologismes et des glossolalies en psychopathologie. Valliant–Carmanne, Liège, 1952.
11. Samarin, W.: Tongues of men and angels, Macmillan, New York, 1972.
12. Laurentin, P.: Pentecôtisme chez les Catholiques: Risques et avenir. Beauchesne, Paris, 1974.
13. Yakovlev, P. I. & Lecours, A. R.: The myelogenetic cycles of regional maturation of the brain. In: A. Minkowski (ed.), Regional Development of the Brain in early Life, p. 3. Blackwell, Oxford and Edinburgh, 1967.
14. Lecours, A. R.: Myelogenetic correlates of the development of speech and language. In: E. H. Lenneberg and E. Lenneberg (eds.), Foundations of Language Development, vol. I, p. 121. Academic Press, New York, 1975.
15. Santerre, L.: Personal communication.
16. Léon, P. & Léon, M.: Introduction à la phonétique corrective. Hachette and Larousse, Paris, 1964.
17. Buyssens, E.: La communication et l'articulation linguistique. Presses Universitaires de Bruxelles and Presses Universitaires de France, Bruxelles and Paris, 1967.
18. Blumstein, S.: A Phonological Investigation of Aphasic Speech. Mouton, the Hague, 1973.
19. Poncet, M., Degos, C., Deloche, G. & Lecours, A. R.: Phonetic and phonemic transformations in aphasia. International Journal of Mental Health 1 (3): 46, 1972.
20. Lecours, A. R., Deloche, G. & Lhermitte, F.: Paraphasies phonémiques: Description et simulation sur ordinateur. In: I.R.I.A. (ed.), Colloques I.R.I.A.: Informatique Médicale, Tome I, p. 311. Institut de Recherche d'Informatique et d'Automatique, Rocquencourt, 1973.
21. Samarin, W.: Personal communication.
22. Christie-Murray, D.: Personal communication.
23. Chaika, E. O.: A linguist looks at 'schizophrenic' language. Brain and Language 1: 257, 1974.
24. Lhermitte, F., Lecours, A. R., Ducarne, B. & Escourolle, R.: Unexpected anatomical findings in a case of fluent jargon aphasia. Cortex 9: 433, 1973.

Reflections on aphasia rehabilitation[1]

ARTHUR BENTON

The central theme of this symposium, so ably organized by Professor Höök and his colleagues, has been aphasia rehabiliation. This does not mean that all the contributions to it have dealt directly with this topic. On the contrary, a number of presentations have considered such fundamental questions as the anatomical and physiopathological bases of aphasic syndromes, the classification of aphasic disorders and the development of methods of diagnostic evaluation. However, all these questions have an important bearing on aphasia rehabilitation for they deal with the basic nature of the conditions that have produced the disabilities which we seek to alleviate.

The persisting problem of the degree of effectiveness of aphasia rehabilitation has been considered in considerable depth and detail. The prevailing tone of the discussion (as reflected, for example, in the analyses of Professor Sarno) has been thoughtful and realistic. No extravagant claims have been made and there is general agreement that at the present time we do not possess specific, definable techniques of predictable effectiveness. This point has been made repeatedly throughout the symposium, particularly by speech therapists who have the most intimate knowledge of the behavioral changes that take place during the course of therapy.

At the same time, the presentations and discussion reflect an extremely important development that has taken place over the past decade. As recently as 10 years ago, there was considerable doubt on the part of many neurologists about whether formal rehabilitation efforts had any effect other than keeping up the aphasic patient's morale. To be sure, there was suggestive evidence that rehabilitation could facilitate recovery, particularly if it was begun as soon as possible and continued over an extended period (3). But as of that time, there had been no unequivocal demonstration that formal language training significantly influenced the rate and degree of restitution of function over and above what might be expected from spontaneous or endogenous recovery (2).

However, over the course of the last 10 years, the findings of a number of studies have indicated that aphasia rehabilitation can facilitate recovery from aphasic disorder. Perhaps the most noteworthy of these investigations is that of the Milan group which has been described by Dr Basso at this Symposium and a preliminary report of which has already been published (1). As a

[1] Concluding remarks at the International Symposium on Aphasia, September 5–8, 1977, Göteborg, Sweden.

consequence, much of the doubt expressed by skeptical neurologists about the value of aphasia rehabilitation has now dissipated.

This encouraging development has generated a large number of specific questions about aphasia rehabilitation, some of which have been considered in depth at this Symposium. For example, if some patients receive significant benefit from therapy, why are other patients not helped? No doubt the personal characteristics of the patient, e.g., age, severity of aphasic disorder, presence of associated cognitive deficits, nature of the underlying neurological condition, account for the failure of treatment in some cases. However, in other cases it may be that inappropriate methods of rehabilitation have been employed, given the particular nature of the impairment in speech and language. The presentations and discussion during the Symposium have made it clear that to answer this and other questions is a most formidable clinical research task. Because of the necessity for counterbalancing the effects of so many determining factors, investigations in this area almost always have to be large in scale. A substantial number of patients have to be evaluated, assigned to different treatment groups, receive treatment over an extended length of time, and be carefully followed through periodic reassessments. The amount of labor required to carry out a simple investigation of this type is prodigious. For example, the study reported by Dr Basso at this Symposium extended over 10 years and involved the combined efforts of a substantial number of neurologists, speech therapists and statisticians.

Professor Sarno has reviewed the many conditions that must be satisfied in order to conduct studies of the effectiveness of aphasia rehabilitation that will yield crucial information about such questions as the type of patient who is likely to benefit from a specific type of therapy, the relative effectiveness of different methods, the optimal time to institute therapy and the point at which therapy should be terminated. One wonders if it is realistic to expect that all these conditions can be satisfied in a single study. Perhaps the most viable approach is to think in terms of a series of carefully planned inter-related collaborative studies of aphasia rehabilitation in a number of centers in different countries. It goes without saying that such a collaborative effort would present its own unique problems and complications. However, given strong central direction, the task could be accomplished, but at a tremendous cost in time, energy and professional talent.

The question that many people will raise is whether costly studies of such magnitude are likely to generate any more meaningful data than have previous studies of a smaller size and a less definitive nature. Some will express doubt that new knowledge of basic importance will be gained even if such studies produce statistically significant findings. They will feel that a more promising approach is to explore new methods of treatment rather than to invest substantial time and labor in determining the extent to which existing methods are effective.

Some of these newer methods of treatment have been described and discussed at the Symposium. Melodic intonation therapy has been reported to be strikingly successful with some non-fluent aphasics. Training in visual communication is effective with some non-speaking patients. The linguistically oriented therapy described by Professor Poeck in his presentation is another example of a highly specific approach which is fitted exactly to a patient's most salient deficits. As Poeck showed, focused therapy, e.g., on a naming disturbance or on agrammatism, can lead to significant and long-lasting improvement, even in patients whose status had not changed over many months. Moreover, the improvement is evident not only in test stituations but in spontaneous speech.

It is important to recognize that the significant ameliorative effects of these newer methods could be demonstrated in very small samples of patients. Large scale studies were not required. In fact, there is much to be said in favor of the principle that, if a specific therapeutic method is truly effective, it should be possible to demonstrate that effectiveness fairly readily with small samples of patients. If a large number of cases is required to arrive at a statistically significant result, there is always an element of doubt about the influence of the specific method as compared to that of numerous other factors in the total situation.

The other path to more effective aphasia rehabilitation is less direct. It consists in enhancing our understanding of the nature of the aphasic disorders and their anatamophysiologic determinants, as exemplified in the experimental and theoretical presentations at the Symposium. Of course, increased knowledge about a pathological condition does not necessarily make it any more treatable or amenable to modification. However, it is reasonable to assume that such knowledge will at least increase the chances of developing rational modes of therapy. Thus these papers are not only of basic importance but also of interest to workers in the field of rehabilitation. For example, the analysis by Professor Sabouraud and his co-workers of the linguistic behavior of a group of patients carrying the diagnostic label of "Broca's aphasia" has specific implications for rehabilitation. If, as they maintain, the fundamental deficit in many of these patients is primarily of a cognitive-linguistic nature and not a disturbance in articulation, it is obvious that the therapeutic approach to these patients must be different from that employed with other patients who carry the same diagnostic label but whose primary difficulty is in articulation.

Thus one sees that proceedings of the Göteborg Symposium on Aphasia have reflected a number of important developments in the field of aphasia rehabilitation. The fact that rehabilitation can facilitate recovery beyond that which would be expected from spontaneous restitution of function has been demonstrated. The encouraging results emerging from the application of innovative treatment methods of a highly specific nature focussed on defined symptoms have been reported and critically discussed. Finally, a number of important contributions to our knowledge of the physiopathology of the aphasic disorders and of their fundamental nature have been presented. These contributions offer the promise that a deeper understanding of aphasia will provide a firmer basis for optimally effective rehabilitation.

References

1. Basso, A., Faglioni, P. & Vignolo, L. A.: Etude controlée de la rééducation du language dans l'aphasie: Comparaison entre aphasiques traités et non-traités. Rev Neurol (Paris) 131: 607, 1975.
2. Benton, A. L. (ed.): Behavioral Change in Cerebrovascular Disease. Harper & Row, New York, 1970.
3. Vignolo, L. A.: Evolution of aphasia and language rehabilitation: A retrospective exploratory study. Cortex 1: 344, 1965.